W.A.I.T.loss

The Keys to Food Freedom
and Winning the Battle of the Binge

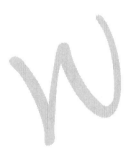

Wendy Hendry

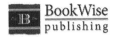

BookWise
publishing

W.A.I.T.*loss*©

The Keys to Food Freedom and Winning the Battle of the Binge

Wendy Hendry

BookWise Publishing

USA

Cover Design by Ida Fla Sveningsson

Book Interior Design by Dayna Linton

Library of Congress Cataloging-in-Publication Data: Pending

W.A.I.T.loss©: The Keys to Food Freedom and Winning the Battle of the Binge

ISBN: (Print version): 978-1-53289-462-6

ISBN: (eBook version): 978-1-60645-153-3

First Printing

10 9 8 7 6 5 4 3 2 1

Praise for W.A.I.T.*loss*

"I love Wendy's book! Her story is warm and funny, and her style is engaging. I couldn't put it down."

—**Ashley Cole,** CEO, Cecelia New York (www.CeceliaNewYork.com)

"If you crave a normal relationship with food, but you're ready to throw in the towel and surrender to a lifetime of obsessing and weighing, **W.A.I.T.** *loss* is the one for you. Wendy's a pro. Listen to her."

—**Sharlene Hawkes,** Miss America 1985, former ESPN Sportscaster, President of RMS Productions

"As a father of seven beautiful daughters, I am well aware of the stress created by weight and body image pressures, especially in women. In her new book, **W.A.I.T.***loss: The Keys to Food Freedom and Winning the Battle of the Binge,* Wendy presents a simple, yet well-researched case for creating healthy habits. She explains it in a way that motivates all to change for the better."

—**David Neeleman,** *Founder, JetBlue Airways*

"Wendy knows her stuff! She has helped many of our challengers lose weight and get happy!" —**Aron Benon,** *CEO of Meltdown Challenge*

"**W.A.I.T.***loss* is invaluable for those who struggle with food addictions and are desperate to be free of them. Wendy is an empathetic, compassionate coach who knows what she's talking about—because she's been there. I highly recommend her book." —**Elayne Wells Harmer,** *Editor/Attorney*

"Not only is **W.A.I.T.***loss* informative and insightful, but Wendy tells of her personal journey which is truly inspiring and motivates and encourages everyone to continue their own journey toward physical and mental health."

—**Sheila B. Hays,** *Clinical Psychologist*

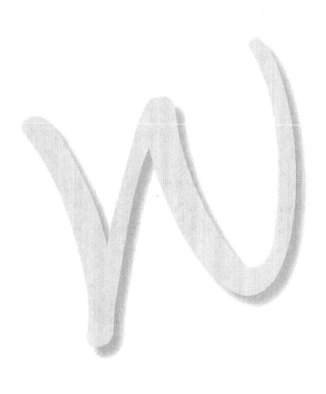

To the hottest husband in the world.
Sorry girls. He's mine.

Table of Contents

Foreword

The weight-loss industry sells the idea that we can achieve our optimal body and perfect health quickly—no waiting involved. But promises of fast results with extreme diets or grueling exercise routines are unrealistic and harmful, especially to those who are prone to binge eating. Binge eating and overeating are widespread among weight-loss dieters and even among those who just want to be healthier. Wendy Hendry saw this all too well in her own life and as a health and nutrition coach—in the life of her clients.

The fact that diets can lead to more binge eating and binge eating can lead to a greater desire to diet makes it easy to see why weight loss and better health seem elusive for some. If binge eaters don't have the right strategies to become healthier and lose weight, they are likely to stay trapped in yo-yo dieting and bingeing cycles, and gain even more weight long term.

Wendy's W.A.I.T.loss© approach offers a way out of this trap and a practical path toward better health.

This book will show you how to get back to basics and wait for the results that will come naturally when you adopt health-giving habits and let go of health-sabotaging ones. Wendy's approach is not just about losing weight; it's about learning how to be in charge of your physical and mental well-being.

I've had the pleasure of knowing Wendy since September of 2014 when an uplifting email popped into my in-box. Wendy said she was almost finished reading my 2011 book, *Brain over Binge*, and she thought it provided a "missing link" in her personal and professional life, in that it could help eliminate a huge roadblock in the journey toward health: binge eating.

Wendy put together so many pieces of the health puzzle before ever encountering my book and even more pieces afterward. Her personal story is inspiring and relatable, and her health advice is no-nonsense. She isn't going to tell you that you have to eat perfectly or follow a set of complicated food rules, but she also isn't going to say that you can overindulge, be sedentary, make poor food choices, and still expect to be healthy.

To the weight-loss industry, this book itself is a powerful "missing link." It bridges the gap for people who are susceptible to binge eating but who also want to lose unhealthy weight and feel their best. It is possible; Wendy and her clients are proof of that.

I'm so glad my book was a part of Wendy's journey, and I know her W.A.I.T.*loss*© approach will be a big part of your own journey toward a healthier life.

—Kathryn Hansen
Author of *Brain over Binge* and *The Brain over Binge Recovery Guide*
March 8, 2016

Self-Evaluation

When I first started my health journey, I did a self-evaluation to determine where my current reality was. I was shocked to take the same evaluation a year later and see how far I had come. I promise if you begin applying the keys here, you will see amazing personal improvement in both your physical and mindful health. Let's start then by focusing on *you*.

I highly encourage you to grab a piece of paper, write down where you are now, and then compare it to where you are in six months or a year from now. Breaking free from any addiction, including food, requires a change in habits, both physical and mental. It takes time for habits to develop, and sometimes the change is gradual. This self-evaluation is a great way for you to see how far you have come. And don't get me wrong. You *will* begin feeling better right away. The thing is as each key principle becomes more firmly entrenched in your brain, your life and health will just keep getting better and better!

1) On a scale of 1 to 5 (5 being wonderful), rate your **physical health**:
How is your weight?
How is your health in general?
Are you taking medications for preventable illnesses?
Do you get daily physical activity?
Do you drink enough water?

2) Using that same scale, rate your **mindful health***:

Do you have time for yourself each day?

How well do you deal with stress?

How many hours do you sleep?

How are your organizational skills?

Do you have a good support system?

3) Lastly, rate your **motivation** to make a change.

*I intentionally use the term *mindful health* over *mental health* as the principles discussed in this book are not about chemical and behavioral disorders. Mindful health is about self-regulation and awareness.

Introduction

This book is not a diet book. Diets do not work! I know this because I'm pretty sure I have tried every diet in the entire world. As a matter of fact, at one time I dieted my way up to about 200 pounds. Diets do the opposite of what we want them to do. Diets make us fat.

What this book does give you are the keys to food freedom! Applying these principles will teach you the habits you need to break free from an unhealthy relationship with food. Most diets have you lose weight with the hope that you will get healthy. This may work short term, but permanent weight loss and optimal health require a permanent change in behavior. By applying the keys to freedom, you will find yourself getting healthier, and the happy consequence will be a healthy weight.

The pinnacle of this book is my W.A.I.T.-and-Click Approach found in the third and final section. I'm sort of an acronym junkie, and W.A.I.T. is an acronym that I developed to help in my own health journey. It stands for—*What Am I Thinking?* W.A.I.T. acts as a cue for us to slow down and take time to breathe. It gives us time to ask if we are actually hungry and if not, to figure out what is triggering the urge. W.A.I.T. is also symbolic. The results of our efforts aren't always immediate, and that's part of the W.A.I.T. It's a reminder of the journey, a request for patience as the path is filled with two steps forward and one step back. The "Click" is the reward, and you will learn all about that in Section 3.

Because I'm so excited about my W.A.I.T.-and-Click Approach, I was tempted to share it at the beginning of the book, as well as The Clicker Club (our support group), but I just couldn't do it. Without the other keys I give you in Sections 1 and 2, the W.A.I.T.-and-Click Approach wouldn't work. I must lay the foundations of physical and mental health in Sections 1 and 2, so you'll be totally set to launch yourself to success with the W.A.I.T.-and-Click Approach in Section 3.

Health comes from having healthy habits. Healthy habits start with motivation to change. Motivation to change starts with us. As soon as we make the decision in our hearts and minds to change, we begin to strengthen ourselves from the inside. This, combined with deepening perseverance, is how we are able to change our habits. By sharing my own personal experiences, as well as what I have learned as a health coach, this book will teach you all of the Keys necessary to find not only good health for your body but also good health for your mind.

I didn't have a normal relationship with my body or with food until I was well into my 40s. Before that my life was filled with a lot of failed diets and frustration. Don't get me wrong. I had a great life. When you don't know what it feels like to feel good, you don't know what you're missing. But once I began to apply the W.A.I.T.*loss*© Keys to physical health explained in Section 1, I began to learn what it feels like to feel good. Once you know that feeling, there is no going back!

Having my physical health is wonderful—I have more stamina. I sleep better and wake earlier. I smile more because I hurt less, and I find myself looking forward to my day instead of dreading it. And yes, I even reached a healthy weight. One problem persisted however. My bingeing did decrease, but it didn't go away. The urges persisted, and the binges continued to take their toll. It wasn't until I learned the Keys to mindful health that the urges *and* the binges started to go away.

My purpose in writing this book is to help you gain that same freedom. It's important to begin giving your body the right nutrition because your mind needs the *exact same fuel.* For this reason, the first section in

W.A.I.T.*loss*©contains the Keys you need to unlock your best physical self. Once you're feeling better physically, your journey to mindful health begins. Section 2 is all about the mind and how we can increase our awareness to conquer the hungry, impetuous part of our brains. Everything I've written is based on scientific studies, which are cited in the Reference Section at the end of this book. Once I've explained each Key, I'll give you a challenge that will help you apply and develop each Key into a habit—that's in Section 3. I promise that as you begin to implement these principles, you will wake up feeling better each day as you discover how wonderful your body can actually feel.

Before we delve into the W.A.I.T.*loss*© specifics, there are a few things that I want to share. First, I want to tell you a little about how my struggle began. Second, I want to share a few facts with you. Third, I'm going to ask you a very important question. Finally, I just want you to know that you're not alone and you *can* take your life back from your urges—and you *can* be free!

—Wendy Hendry

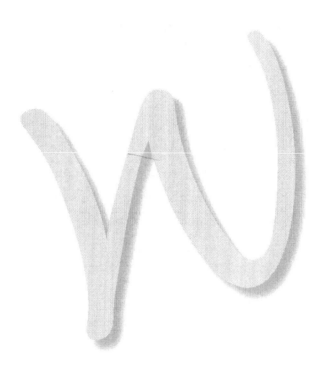

Wendy's Story

Part 1: The Cycle Begins

My addiction started at a liquor store, which is ironic as it has nothing to do with alcohol.

Vic's Liquor Store was where my dad sent my brother and me when we came home early one day and saw him packing his bags. I asked him where he was going, and he responded, "Here's some money. Go buy some candy at Vic's. I'll meet you there." My brother was ten, and I was twelve. I'm pretty sure that we both understood at the time that this trek to Vic's was going to be bittersweet.

As we walked out of Vic's with our bags of Tootsie Rolls and Pixy Stix and the gum that looked like cigarettes and even blew white confectionery smoke, my dad pulled up and told us that he was moving out and divorcing my mom. He was crying when he told us, and I had never seen him cry. He had to get to work, so he kissed us goodbye, and Greg and I walked home. I'm not sure what Greg did once we got home, but I went straight to my room and ate my whole bag of candy. Tootsie Rolls helped me forget that my dad wasn't coming home after work anymore.

I don't mean to share my story for sympathy or pity, but knowing when and how my jail sentence with food started will help explain how I was finally set free.

Vic's candy aisle became my favorite afternoon venue. I would sneak into my mom's wallet and take her cash and then stop at Vic's on the way home from school, hiding the candy under my pillow to eat at night. Food was my counselor, my priest, and my best friend all rolled into one. It never occurred to me that what I was doing was bad or unhealthy.

I didn't really think about my health or my weight, at least until tenth grade. That was when we were required to take social studies. My teacher, Mr. Tedman, was big and bald, except for the horseshoe of red hair around the bottom of his head. His class was right after lunch, and my friend, Dana, and I would often take food into his class to eat. Mr. Tedman was relentless in his comments to Dana and me about our weight. Every day he would tease us—saying that we were fat or that we shouldn't be eating this or that. We endured that the entire year. We each gained twenty to thirty pounds during that school year, bringing us both close to around 150 pounds, which was heavy for my 5-foot 3-inch frame.

Over the summer, Dana and I decided that we were both going to go on diets. We made a plan, and then I left for Utah to spend the summer with my dad. My plan was that I would allow myself half a sandwich and a piece of fruit each day. For a treat, I could have a cup of hot chocolate (my dad worked at a market where they had one of those hot chocolate machines). By the time summer ended, I was down to around 115 pounds.

When I came home and walked off the plane, my mom was not happy with what she saw. I insisted I was fine and probably gave her that "leave-me-alone scowl" that my teenagers now give to me. The next week I saw Dana at church. She was even thinner than I was. Once school started, I allowed myself a half of an egg salad sandwich and an apple each day. I lost a little bit more weight, but Dana wasn't eating anything, and she was starting to look really bad.

One day my mom said, "You're starting to look like Dana." She knew I wasn't eating either. Luckily, I could see what would happen if I stayed on that path. I think I was also looking for an excuse to start eating, and eat I did! By the time I graduated, I was bigger than ever, and food began to consume my thoughts more and more.

A Few Facts

Fact: No country has successfully reduced its rate of obesity since 1982. **(0.1)**

Fact: Since 1980 the obesity rate has more than doubled.

Fact: Being overweight cannot only impact your health, it can kill you.

Fact: Obesity can be prevented. **(0.2)**

Fact: Two out of three people in America are overweight.

Fact: More than one-third of Americans are in the obese category (BMI greater than or equal to 30). **(0.3)**

Fact: By 2030 it's estimated that 42 percent of Americans will be obese. The report also predicts that the proportion of Americans who are severely obese (over 100 pounds overweight) will double to 11 percent. **(0.4)**

Fact: W.A.I.T.loss© contains the solution to this scary trend.

Big is Beautiful, Sort of

Since becoming a health coach, I have had a few people say to me that I'm doing a disservice to people because I'm perpetuating the idea that big is not beautiful. My response—beauty has nothing to do with it. Someone told me once that it's not about the dress size. It's about what's in the dress.

It took me a long time to admit that obesity is not a skin-deep problem. As a matter of fact, I spent years preaching that big is beautiful. The problem is that being overweight can put us at higher risk for type 2 diabetes, coronary heart disease, stroke, cancer, sleep apnea, metabolic syndrome, reproductive problems, arthritis, etc. So even though big can be beautiful on the outside, if we want to feel good and be healthy, we need to watch the scale.

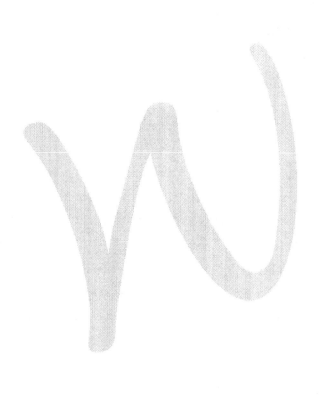

Wendy's Story

From Pixy Stix to Sweaty Chix™

By the time I was 36 and done having kids, my weight peaked at about 200 pounds. I couldn't walk around the block without huffing and puffing. I decided that I wanted to start exercising. I joined the gym and fell in love with the kick-boxing classes.

After about a year, my weight had dropped to 150 pounds, and I was proudly sporting a size 12/13. I felt pretty good about myself and decided that I wanted to be a fitness instructor. I became certified as a kick-boxing instructor and set out to find a class to teach. It wasn't long before I realized that the gyms liked their fitness instructors to be size XS and still in diapers.

After several condescending looks, I decided, *Screw the gyms,* and I started my own classes. My very first class started as a freebie at my church and had two people. Skip ahead six years and I'm running my own fitness business called Sweaty Chix Fitness™. I hired about twelve other instructors, and we taught about fifty or so classes each week.

My mission at Sweaty Chix™ was "Exercise at any size." I really wanted Sweaty Chix™ to be for the women that didn't feel comfortable in the gym atmosphere, and I'm proud of the fact that it became just that. I preached in my classes that our weight didn't matter as long as we felt good and were happy. I really did believe that, but mostly I wanted my Chix to feel good about themselves. Size just wasn't an issue in my classes. We were just a group of friends trying to break a sweat every day.

Sweaty Chix™ was good for me too because surrounding myself with like-minded women helped me come to a place of acceptance of my weight. I really didn't pay as much attention to the scale as long as I was active every day. After some time though I noticed my clothes were getting tighter, and I was surprised when I stepped on the scale to be back up to 170 pounds.

It was about this time that I went to the doctor for a routine checkup. Except for the shock of stepping on the scale, I felt pretty good. After the poking and prodding, my doctor told me that my cholesterol was high, my blood pressure was high, and that I would probably end up with diabetes if I didn't lose some weight. When I asked him how that could be since I exercised every day, he explained, "Well, you probably eat too much." Being told that I needed to lose weight did slap the pride out of me, but it didn't make me change my "weight doesn't matter" philosophy.

It wasn't until a few months later that I did a complete turnaround in my thinking. It was the day after Thanksgiving 2012, and my mom had just had a stroke. My mom was a wonderful, talented, lovely woman, but she spent the majority of her life morbidly obese. After her stroke she couldn't walk. It took three people and a lift machine to help her out of bed. She hated it, and so did I.

I watched my mom go from a happy, self-sufficient woman to an embarrassed and highly dependent invalid. I feel guilty about it now, but while she was in the nursing home, I was angry with her. I was angry because I knew she had put herself in that position by allowing herself to be overweight. I kept thinking that had she exercised more or eaten less, she would still be walking. The more I watched her deteriorate, the angrier I became.

I can't remember the exact moment that it happened, but eventually I realized that I wasn't angry with her. I was angry with myself. Even though I was a fitness instructor, I was not taking care of my body. It hit me that if I didn't change something, I was going to end up in a nursing home just like my sweet mom. She died five months after her stroke.

The moral of this story is that our opinions on the "big is beautiful" issue are irrelevant. No matter how good we look in a size XXL, the cons of being overweight outweigh (no pun intended) the pros. The only way we can reverse the obesity epidemic is to start with ourselves.

Thankfully, I was able to get healthy, and now I know how good that feels. *That* is the reason I wrote this book. I want you to know how *good* health feels. I'm hoping that the principles we talk about will ignite a fire inside of you to get healthy. Then I hope you will go ignite that same fire in others by teaching them the things that you have learned.

The Important Question

Motivation is always fueled by a "why," and some "whys" are more effective than others. For example, when I was in high school, I started working as a waitress. I wanted to have money to buy clothes and extra stuff. Not long after I started working, my mom lost her job. My motivation to work became much greater as her need for help with the bills increased. Motivation based on temporary, superficial "whys," like buying clothes, is *Lower Level* motivation. *Higher Level* motivation is based on broader, longer-reaching, selfless "whys."

Another example can be found in the Navy. In order to become a Navy Seal, candidates must pass through a boot camp called *Hell Week* that is more like torture than training. It's five-and-half days of brutal physical drills that test physical endurance, mental toughness, and determination. The candidates do this on less than four hours of sleep, and only one in four makes it through to the end. It has been noted that the 25 percent of those who survive *Hell Week* are not necessarily those with the biggest muscles. The ones who succeed are those with the *Higher Level* motivators.

Eric Greitens, a SEAL officer recalling his fellow *Hell Week* survivors noted, "They had the ability to step outside of their own pain, put aside their own fear and ask, 'How can I help the guy next to me?' They had more than the 'fist' of courage and physical strength. They also had a heart large enough to think about others." **(0.5,0.6)**

The *Highest Level* "whys" are those that consider others. I've found that my clients who want to get healthy for their kids or their spouses have much more success than those who want to lose a few pounds to fit into a pair of skinny jeans. So when considering your "why," try to focus it on the *Higher Level*.

W.A.I.T.*loss* Challenge:

Make a list of the things that are driving your motivation to get healthy. Mark the ones that are higher level.

Section 1: W.A.I.T.
Physical Freedom

Becoming a **W.A.I.T.loss**© pro means that you apply *"What Am I Thinking?"*—self-awareness—to every aspect of your life. As far as your nutritional health is concerned, applying W.A.I.T. means that eventually you will become an intuitive eater. Intuitive eating* means allowing your own internal voice to dictate when, what, and how much we should eat. The problem for those of us who struggle with food issues is that we've lost our internal voice. Section 1 will help you find that again.

The ability to perceive our internal physiological cues, including hunger, is what scientists call *interoception*. In a perfect world, we would all have goof-proof interoception. However, if you're anything like I was, it's been a long time since you could tell the difference between hunger, cravings, anxiety, boredom, and a Twinkie. The good news is that we can fix that. We can undo the damage that years of messed-up diets and restriction have done to our brains. The first step is to fake an unimpaired interoception until it becomes the real deal. In other words, we need to go back to the baby steps and train our body *when* to eat, *what* to eat, and *how* to eat. **(1.1,1.2)**

One thing to keep in mind as you make these changes is that everyone's body is different. Most people will start feeling better as soon as they start making changes, but for others, it takes a while for the body to adjust. Sometimes the first few days can be rough because you're adjusting to healthier foods and ridding the body of inflammation and toxins that come with eating the wrong foods. Some of my clients have reported migraines, nausea, flu-like symptoms, etc. Don't let that catch you off guard. *Push through!*

*Intuitive eating doesn't necessarily mean it's a free-for-all. I will address "restrictive" eating later in the book, but for now understand that intuition and restriction are not mutually exclusive.

Key #1: WHEN to Eat
The Grazing Approach

I'm assuming that many of you reading this book understand the agony that comes with not being able to pull your pants up over your thighs. You may have, like me, felt the shame of shopping at the "fat lady" store or delicately holding a piece of celery at a party instead of the cheesecake because someone might be watching. Maybe, like me, you have given up applying makeup because you think you are beyond help. I hated those feelings, and it makes me sad to think of all of the people who are waking up each day to those same emotions.

I understand personally why the diet industry brought in $64 billion last year in this country alone. Between the time I was 12 and 45, I did every diet imaginable—*South Beach, Weight Watchers, Atkins, Nutrisystem, Paleo, HCG, Grapefruit,* and many more, some of which I invented myself. I absolutely dieted myself into obesity.

A typical day of non-diet eating in my life looked something like this:

Breakfast: What's breakfast?

Lunch: "Healthy" fruit and fro-yo smoothie, and a big piece of "healthy" bread from the neighborhood bakery.

Dinner: Whatever I could get my hands on because I was starving.

Beyond Dinner: Whatever I could get my hands on because—what the he$$—I've already messed up, and I'll start a diet tomorrow.

There really was no consistency to my eating patterns, except to say that they were consistently messed up. It was pretty much a binge-restrict cycle until I discovered the Key Principles I outline in this book.

The very first thing that I learned was how important it is to eat every two to three hours. Initially, I could not comprehend eating that often without gaining weight. I only tried it because of a recommendation from a friend who was also a health coach, and I'm sure glad I did! After less than a week of eating every few hours, I noticed that I had a lot more energy and a lot less naps. Not only did eating on a regular basis give me more stamina, by the end of week one, I had lost five pounds.

Since that time, I have seen hundreds of people convert to "grazing." Personally, I'm sold, and for the most part, science backs me up. Research has shown that those who "nibble" have lower body weights than those who eat few and larger meals. Other studies have shown that irregular meal patterns may also eventually lead to obesity and that regular meal times may actually lead to weight loss. **(1.3, 1.4)**

One way to put it into perspective is to compare your body to a car. Is there any way to put enough gas into your car to drive from California to New York? As far as I know, there are no cars that can make 3,000 miles on one tank of gas. You have to fill it as you go. Your body's "gas tank" is the same way. It wasn't made to hold enough "fuel" to get you all the way to New York. Your "engine" needs to refuel along the way too. **(1.5)**

I have seen with my own eyes the benefits of eating smaller, more frequent meals, but I wanted some extra "real-world" proof. So I sent out a survey to over 1,000 women asking about their eating habits. My very unscientific approach overwhelmingly supported the "grazing" method. A whopping 70 percent of those whose BMI fell in the healthy range considered themselves "grazers." **(1.6)**

Not only does eating smaller meals throughout the day reduce obesity, it also reduces heart disease, improves cholesterol, and stabilizes blood sugar. **(1.7)**

Another affirmation to grazing is pure common sense. Being hungry leads to bingeing. Even though our brain does at times throw out urges to binge because of non-hunger-related triggers, many times bingeing is the result of hunger. When we let ourselves get hungry, we have a tendency to want to eat way too much of the wrong things. Eating every few hours not only helps with satiety, but it also gives us a little something to look forward to. Even as I sit here typing, I can focus on my work instead of food because 1) I ate only an hour ago, so my tummy isn't rumbling, and 2) I know I don't have to wait until tonight to eat. I'll be nibbling again on something yummy in a couple of hours. **(1.8)**

W.A.I.T.*loss* Challenge:

Set a timer to eat every two to three hours. Do this all day long, and don't be afraid to eat a little before bedtime. Do NOT go over three hours without fueling your body. I know this is a scary concept for many people. It was for me! This is how you train your body to do what it is meant to do. If you still are hesitant, just remember that what you are doing now isn't working, so trust this new system and see if it doesn't work miracles for you like it did for me. And please read on—I'm going to give you even more guidance, so you'll feel secure, educated, and empowered in doing this and every one of the W.A.I.T.loss challenges!

Key #2: WHEN to Eat
Don't Skip Breakfast

The first part of fueling your body like a Smart Car is eating breakfast. You wouldn't want to start out your trip across country with an empty tank! Eating breakfast was a difficult concept for me because I was so used to bingeing after the first bite of the day. In my head, I thought that eating early would just start out my bingeing that much sooner. However, I realized right away that bingeing in the morning wasn't a problem. I didn't understand why at the time, but I know now that it's because our willpower is naturally stronger in the mornings. We will discuss this further in Section 2.

One thing I've learned is that the body will pretty much adapt to whatever we teach it. I had been avoiding breakfast for so long that my body was just used to not eating it. Part of my challenge was retraining my body to do the healthy thing. This is the "faked" interoception that I wrote about earlier. Faking it proved successful as it didn't take much time at all for my body to tell me on its own that an early morning meal was surely needed.

Studies have shown that people who eat breakfast have:

- Lower BMIs
- Better memory and cognitive performance
- Less risk of coronary heart disease
- Less hunger throughout the day

- Increased daily fiber consumption
- Less risk of type 2 diabetes **(1.9, 1.10, 1.11)**

Breakfast is also important because it restores the blood glucose level to normal and signals to the body that the overnight fast is over. This is important as glucose is the body's main energy source. Another little breakfast perk is that it reduces the nightly production of cortisol. We'll talk about that in a later chapter, but trust me. That's a good thing. **(1.12)**

W.A.I.T *loss* Challenge:

Eat within 30 minutes of waking up. This can be especially challenging if you overindulged the night before. Do NOT be deterred! In order to train your body to do the right thing, you have to stay the course. If you binged the night before and then skip breakfast the next morning, you're more likely to binge again that night. In order to break the cycle, you have to get out of the binge-restrict cycle, even if that means working on the "no restrict" part first.

Key #3: WHAT to Eat
The 3 Macro-Nutrients

We live on a half-acre. That's a lot of grass to mow. At least that's what my teenage sons tell me when I force them to mow it. Because my husband and I are such nice parents, we decided to buy a riding lawn mower for them to use. We hadn't had the lawn mower for very long when our sweet boys decided to surprise us and mow the lawn without coercion. The mower was out of gas, so they (the boys) found a gas can in the shed and filled up the tank. Unfortunately, that gas can was filled with a gas/oil mixture that my husband had prepared up for our tiller. Apparently you can't use the wrong fuel and expect a John Deere to run smoothly. That was an expensive "surprise."

Using the right fuel is not only vital where John Deere lawn mowers are concerned. Nourishing your body on the proper fuel is the only way to keep your "motor" running efficiently as well. Thankfully, you don't need to drink gasoline for energy. Instead, your body uses carbohydrates, proteins, and fats.

> **CAUTION:**
> I'm getting ready to throw a bunch of nutritional information at you. Don't let it put you on the crazy train. Use this section to refer back to on an as needed basis. I'll teach you how to make this easy later. You can also check out my secret weapon in the simple tips section that follows.

Carbohydrates

The gasoline that we use to fuel cars is a byproduct of crude oil. In similar fashion, the fuel our bodies use for energy is a byproduct of carbohydrates. This fuel is a type of sugar called glucose and is our body's preferred source of energy. Glucose provides quick and readily available energy. Have you ever heard of "carb-loading"? Before endurance athletes have to perform, they fuel with extra carbs so that their muscles will be filled with glucose, i.e., readily available energy.

Another reason we need carbs is because the human brain is also fueled by glucose. So if we want to think, remember, and learn things, we need to keep some "gas" in our brains. (We will talk more about our brain chemistry in Section 2.) Also, because carbs contain fiber, they help reduce that icky, bloated feeling by keeping the bowels moving. Carbs also contain vitamins and can help reduce cholesterol. Personally, my favorite reason for eating carbs is because they just taste good. **(1.13)**

Carbs have been getting a bad rap over the last few decades, but our bodies wouldn't go very far without them. Most carbs are broken down into glucose. Glucose is a fancy name for sugar. Once the sugar gets into the bloodstream, it signals to the body to produce a hormone called insulin. I won't get into the details about the role of insulin, but I will say that too much of it is bad for us and can eventually cause serious illnesses, such as diabetes and heart disease.

This sort of puts the body into a deadlock. We need carbs to function, yet carbs can eventually lead to obesity and illness. Luckily there is a solution to this predicament. We can give our bodies fuel and avoid the disadvantages by choosing the *right* carbohydrates.

LOW GI (less than or equal to 55)		High GI (56+)	
FOOD	GI	FOOD	GI
Cauliflower	6	White Rice	56
Lettuce	7	Pita Bread	56
Broccoli	10	Wild Rice	57
Onions	10	Blueberry Muffin	57
Spinach	12	Mango	59
Peanuts	14	Couscous	60
Walnuts	15	Pancakes	61
Green Beans	15	Raisins	63
Pearled Barley	22	Pineapple	64
Cherries	22	Angel Food Cake	66
Cashews	22	Croissant	67
Plums	24	Whole Wheat	67
Grapefruit	25	Bread	68
Kidney Beans	27	Plum	69
Peaches	28	White Bread	70
Lentils	29	Corn Tortilla	70
Egg Fettuccine	32	Watermelon	72
Apples	34	Corn Chips	72
Yogurt, Plain	36	Mashed Potatoes	73
Ice Cream	38	Graham Cracker	74
Tomato	38	Pumpkin	75
Pinto Beans	39	Donuts	75
Green Peas	39	Vanilla Wafers	77
Strawberries	40	Jelly Beans	78
Milk, Whole	40	Gatorade	78
Grapes	43	Carrots, Cooked	80
Soy Milk	44	Crackers	80
Orange	48	Rice Cakes	82
Brown Rice	50	Pretzels	83
Banana	51	Baked Potato	85
Mango	51	Carrot, Raw	92
Sweet Potato	54	Fruit Roll-ups	98
Oatmeal	55	Dates	100
White Pasta	55		
Corn, Yellow	55		

Fruits, vegetables, nuts, and other foods have "good," "better," and "best" gradients in regards to sugar content. Some carbs put more sugar, and therefore more insulin, into the bloodstream than others. The actual impact of carbohydrates on blood sugar is gauged by a measurement called the glycemic index (GI). Previously, foods were analyzed by their carbohydrate count (grams per serving). The GI value measures instead the impact of foods on blood sugar. In other words, the higher the GI value, the more sugar that particular food will put into your body. Most organizations rank sugar content using a "high" and "low" rating system.

Proteins

It's true that "Man shall not live on bread [and other carbs] alone." (Matt 4:4) It's important that we balance out our carbohydrates with other nutrients, such as proteins. Proteins are made up of smaller compounds called amino acids, also known as the body's building blocks. When we eat proteins, the body breaks them down into amino acids. These tiny building blocks are then built back up into different structures, such as muscles, hormones, body organs, antibodies, tissues, and many other things that are essential to the body.

Another important function, albeit secondary, of protein is to provide energy. Although protein isn't the body's main source of energy, it can be converted to glucose when needed. This is another reason why it's important to have carbohydrates in our diets. If we don't have enough carbs in our system, the body breaks down some of our lean muscle mass for energy.

Dr. Dan Benardot explains this further in his book *Nutrition for Serious Athletes*:

A standard tenet in nutrition is that carbohydrates have a protein-sparing effect. What this really means is that if you can supply sufficient carbohydrates to the system for fuel, then protein will be spared from being burned and used for more important functions. **(1.14)**

Most of the time protein brings to mind chicken, beef, and fish, but there are lots of great and surprising sources of protein, such as hemp seeds (1/4 cup = 13 g), edamame (1 cup in pod = 8 g), Greek yogurt (1 cup = 24 g), ricotta cheese (1/2 cup = 14 g), and eggs (1 egg = 6 g).

Some of My Favorite Proteins

MEAT	DAIRY PROTEIN	VEGAN OPTIONS
Chicken Breast, Skinless	Swiss Cheese	Tofu
Turkey Breast	Cottage Cheese	Edamame
Lean Ground Turkey	Egg Whites	Wheat Germ
Swordfish	Eggs	Quinoa
Orange Roughy	Egg Substitutes	Green Peas
Haddock	Whey Protein Powder	White Beans
Salmon	Greek Yogurt	Pinto Beans
Tuna	Ricotta Cheese	Black Beans
Crab	Mozzarella Cheese	Chickpeas
Lobster		Leafy Greens
Shrimp		Navy Beans
Top Round Steak		Lentils
Top Sirloin Steak		Amaranth
Extra Lean Ground Beef		Peanut Butter
Halibut		Mixed Nuts
Tilapia		

Some foods are naturally nutrient balanced. For example, one cup of quinoa contains 39 grams of carbs and 8 grams of protein. One cup of lentils has 40 grams of carbs and 14 grams of protein. One cup of almonds has 20 grams of carbs and 20 grams of protein.

You don't have to limit yourself to things on a list though. You can generally find all of the info you need right on a food's nutrition label. It's important to get into the habit of reading the nutrition label before you put a food item in your grocery basket.

Recent studies have shown that it's essential to get in enough protein, but it's also important to pay attention to how and when you eat it. Spreading your protein intake throughout the day will allow your body to continue maintaining its muscle mass.

Also, having protein at each meal helps with satiety because protein is digested much more slowly than carbohydrates. Have you noticed that when you eat an orange or a piece of bread, you're hungry a few minutes later? Protein will keep you satisfied for much longer. I always recommend to my clients that they pair a protein with their carbs. If they are going to eat a donut, I tell them to have some chicken or cottage cheese or another protein with it. (Of course it would be better if they picked a low glycemic carb!) Adding in some protein will help you consume less of the "bad" carbs also. **(1.15,1.16)**

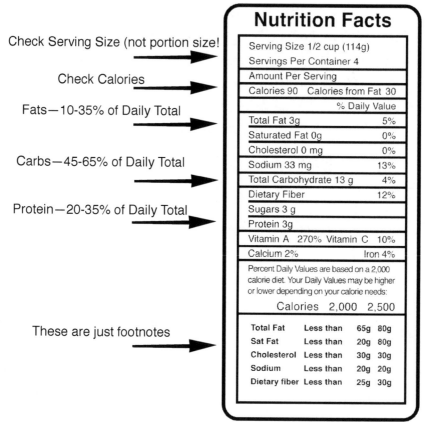

Check Serving Size (not portion size!

Check Calories

Fats—10-35% of Daily Total

Carbs—45-65% of Daily Total

Protein—20-35% of Daily Total

These are just footnotes

Nutrition Facts

Serving Size 1/2 cup (114g)
Servings Per Container 4

Amount Per Serving	
Calories 90 Calories from Fat 30	
	% Daily Value
Total Fat 3g	5%
Saturated Fat 0g	0%
Cholesterol 0 mg	0%
Sodium 33 mg	13%
Total Carbohydrate 13 g	4%
Dietary Fiber	12%
Sugars 3 g	
Protein 3g	
Vitamin A 270% Vitamin C 10%	
Calcium 2% Iron 4%	

Percent Daily Values are based on a 2,000 calorie diet. Your Daily Values may be higher or lower depending on your calorie needs:

Calories	2,000	2,500
Total Fat	Less than	65g	80g
Sat Fat	Less than	20g	80g
Cholesterol	Less than	30g	30g
Sodium	Less than	20g	20g
Dietary fiber	Less than	25g	30g

Fats

Fat sounds like something that we would not want to purposefully consume. Our generation was raised to believe that low-fat diets are the best way to lose weight. When we look at the increased obesity over the last forty years, it should be obvious that the low-fat diet theory hasn't been working. Over the last several years, science has backed up what has been obvious on the scales. I read through over twenty credible clinical studies that compared weight loss with low-carb versus low-fat diets. Every single one came up with the same conclusion: low-carb diets are more effective for weight loss than low-fat diets. Several of these studies also suggested that those on low-carb diets saw decreased cholesterol and insulin levels as well as significantly reduced hunger.

Conclusion: Fat is not the enemy! It is not only vital to our survival, but it helps us stay trim and healthy.

Fats function as one of the most practical and ingenious parts of our entire body. When you understand its purpose, you will realize that fat is our friend, not our foe. Fat is our food storage system! What happens when a car runs out of gas, and there is no gas station close by? Of course, it stops running. Fat prevents that from happening to us. It's like a portable gas station that we carry with us!

Along with emergency energy, fat also acts as the body's insulator, keeping us warm in the winter and cool in the summer. Fat also keeps our hair and skin soft and the digestive system running smoothly.

Why is it that fat so often has a negative association? Obviously, too much stored fat can be unhealthy, but there are some consumable fats that we need to avoid also. Just like with carbs, there are the good guys and the bad guys.

Trans Fats: The Bad Guys

There is a lot of debate in the nutrition world, but one thing that scientists do agree on is that trans fats should be avoided. There is a type of natural trans fat that can be found in some meat and dairy products, but this is not the one that you need to steer clear of. Artificial trans fats are a different story. Artificial trans fats, also called hydrogenated fats, are a byproduct of a process that turns liquid fat into solid. It's generally used as a preservative. Not only do these fats increase your risk for heart disease, but also some studies suggest that they may raise your risk of type 2 diabetes. Trans fats increase inflammation in overweight and obese people and can damage the lining of blood vessels. As if these things weren't enough, there is also evidence that they may also increase the risk of cancer. Bottom line is, avoid trans fats! If a food label has the words "hydrogenated" or "partially hydrogenated" on the ingredients list, treat it like the poison that it is, and stay far, *far* away. **(1.17)**

Saturated Fats: The Undetermined

Saturated fats are the ones that we use most often in this country. It has generally been accepted as fact that too much saturated fat can raise cholesterol and increase the chances of heart disease. But recently studies have been done that question that longtime theory. These studies concluded that there was not enough evidence to support the claim that saturated fats definitely increase the risk of heart disease. **(1.18)** Even with this evidence, most medical professionals, including the American Heart Association, recommend that healthy people limit the amount of saturated fats to less than 7 percent of their total daily calories. For those who need to lower their cholesterol, they recommend even lower levels, 5 to 6 percent. **(1.19)**

Saturated fats can be found in many of our everyday foods, especially meat products, including beef, pork, poultry skin, lamb, etc. Saturated fats are also found in butter, lard, cheese, and other dairy products.

Unsaturated Fats: The Good Guys

In 1956, Ancel Keys, a researcher at the University of Minnesota, set out to examine the epidemic of heart attacks in middle-aged American men. His theory was that this plague was related to their lifestyle and physicality. Eventually, the study included other countries and became known as the Seven Countries Study. The countries included Greece, Yugoslavia, Finland, the Netherlands, Italy, Japan, and the United States. Keys and his comrades explored the lifestyle habits, diet, and heart disease prevalence from each of these regions. They discovered that despite their high-fat diet, the people in Greece had less heart disease than in other parts of the world. The reason, they concluded, was because the fat used in Mediterranean food was olive oil. **(1.20)**

Olive oil is an unsaturated fat. Unlike saturated fats, unsaturated fats are liquid at room temperature, and besides olive oil they include canola oil and peanut oil. They are also found in nuts and avocados. Omega fats, which are found in fish, eggs, lean meat, soybeans, walnuts, sunflower seeds, sesame oils, etc., are also unsaturated and should be eaten daily.

FATS IN FOODS		
High in Unsaturated Fats	High in Saturated Fats	High in Trans Fats
Canola Oil	Butter	Lard
Olive Oil	Cream	Vegetable Shortening
Avocado	Whole Milk	Most Margarines
Nuts (Almonds, Cashews, etc.)	Cheese	Donuts
Egg Yolk	Ice Cream	Muffins
Safflower Oil	Chocolate	Pies
Fish and Fish Oils	Coconuts	Fast Foods
Most Vegetable Oils	Red Meat	Other Things That Are Happy

Image Copyright 2016 BookWise Publishing LLC

These "good" fats are like the "lube" oil in your engine! They can actually improve cholesterol levels and lower your risk of heart disease by 15 to 25 percent. They have even been shown to control blood sugar and may also help with insulin levels.

These healthy fats should make up most of your daily fat intake. **(1.21)**

W.A.I.T *loss* Challenge:

Start to get in the habit of pairing a protein with a carb every time you eat. We will break it down into specifics next, but for now, just make sure that each meal has some protein.

Bonus Challenge:

You can also begin to read the nutrition labels on your food.

Key #4: How Much to Eat
Portions and PROportions

Honestly, I really struggled with this part of the book. There are two things that I hate in life. One is counting calories, and the other is stepping on the scale. I couldn't decide if I even wanted to include any of that as I really wanted this book to be more about mindfulness and overcoming urges. However, if you're not feeding your body correctly, it's pretty much impossible to work on the cognitive part of things. So I made an executive decision. I decided to include a calorie chart as you do need to know about how much to eat, but I'm leaving out the weight and BMI charts. I want your focus to be on feeling your best. The healthy weight will come naturally.

The number of calories each person needs depends on several factors, including age, gender, height, and activity level. Another important component includes what you want to achieve. Do you want to lose weight? Gain weight? Maintain your current weight? The following recommendations are from the Dietary Guidelines for Americans, but remember that these are only estimates.

Side note: the best way to regulate your individual caloric needs is to keep an eye on your own health and weight, and monitor accordingly. (1.22)

ESTIMATED CALORIE NEEDS PER DAY BY AGE, GENDER, AND PHYSICAL ACTIVITY LEVEL[a]				
		PHYSICAL ACTIVITY		
GENDER	AGE (YEARS)	SEDENTARY	MODERATELY ACTIVE	ACTIVE
Child (female & male)	2-3	1000-2000[b]	1000-1400[c]	1000-1400[c]
Female[d]	4-8	1200-1400	1400-1600	1400-1600
	9-13	1400-1600	1600-2000	1600-2000
	14-18	1800	2000	2400
	19-30	1800-2000	2000-2200	2400
	31-50	1800	2000	2200
	51+	1600	1800	2000-2200
Male	4-8	1200-1400	1400-1600	1600-2000
	9-13	1600-2000	1800-2200	2000-2600
	14-18	2000-2400	2400-2800	2800-3000
	19-30	2400-2600	2400-2600	3000
	31-50	2200-2400	2200-2400	2800-3000
	51+	2000-2200	2200-2400	2400-2800

a. Based on estimated energy requirements (EER) equations using reference heights (average) and reference weights (healthy) for each age/gender group. For children and adolescents, reference height and weight vary. For adults, the reference man is 5 feet 10 inches tall and weighs 154 pounds. The reference woman is 5 feet 4 inches tall and weighs 126 pounds. EER equations are from the Institute of Medicine Dietary Reference intakes for Energy, Carbohydrates, Fiber, Fat, Fatty Acids, Cholesterol, Protein, and Amino Acids, Washington (DC): The National Academics Press; 2002.
b. Sedentary means a lifestyle that includes only the light physical activity associated with typical day-to-day life. Moderately active means a lifestyle with physical activity equivalent to walking 1.5 to 3 miles per day at 3 to 4 miles per hour. In addition to the light physical activity associated with typical day-to-day life.
c. The calorie ranges shown are to accommodate needs of different ages within the group. For children and adolescents, more calories are needed at older ages. For adults, fewer calories are needed at older ages.
d. Estimates for females do not include women who are pregnant or breastfeeding.

If you're anything like me, eating 2,000 calories is an uneasy notion. Unless I was bingeing, I was used to eating far less. (That's why I was bingeing!) When I did start eating the amount of food suggested, I was surprised that I could eat that much and lose weight. I continue to be surprised at how much I can eat and maintain. Many of my clients are obese because they do *not* eat enough. You have to eat to be healthy, but you also have to eat right. Remember the goal is to put your body on cruise control using the right fuel.

Portion Distortion

It's not a secret that portion sizes have increased significantly since the 1980s. Not even the Quarter Pounder® is a quarter pound anymore! Bagels have gone from 3-inch diameters to 6-inch diameters. Chinese takeout has gone from a half-pint to a quart container. A serving of French fries used to be 2.4 ounces. Now the average is 6.9 ounces. That's a difference of 400 calories! Even the average coffee has increased from 45 to 350 calories. You get the point. The hard reality, however, is that portion size is *not* the reason the obesity rate has more than doubled in the same amount of time. The reason obesity has increased is because we are *eating* those bigger portions.

One thing that needs to be stressed is that even though portion sizes have increased dramatically, serving sizes have not. Portion size is how much we *actually* eat. Serving size is how much we *should* eat. Sometimes the difference between serving size and portion size is considerable. Serving sizes are listed on the nutrition label. The problem is that people check the nutrition labels for calories, but they don't realize that they need to check the serving size as well. Mistaking serving size for portion size is what gets us in trouble and is referred to by many as "portion distortion." For example, those little pints of premium ice cream can easily be one *portion size* for most people, including myself. But in reality they contain four *serving sizes*!

Before I understood serving sizes, I looked at the calories and assumed my portion, the pint container, was 260 calories. Nope. There is actually a whopping 1,040 calories in that deceitful little carton. No wonder I was 200 pounds!

I grew up down the street from a 7-Eleven. I remember the arrival of the 32-ounce Big Gulp®. It was a big deal! When my mom was young, a large soft drink was 7 ounces. So even though in my mind, that 32-ounce Big Gulp was one portion, it actually contained more than four servings. Now you can buy 128 ounces of Gulp. That's a full gallon or almost twenty 7-ounce servings! And the average stomach only holds 30 ounces!

Here's an example of some other common serving sizes that may surprise you. For each of the following, note what the single serving size equals:

- 1 slice of bread (so a sandwich has two servings of bread)
- ½ cup cooked rice or pasta (most restaurants serve 2 cups or 4 servings)
- 1 pancake (about the size of your hand)
- 1 small piece of fruit (about the size of your fist)
- ½ cup fruit juice (most small bottles of juice have more so read the label)
- 1 cup of milk or yogurt
- 1 teaspoon of margarine (about the size of half your thumb)
- ½ cup of ice cream (about the size of a baseball)
- 2 ounces of cheese (about the size of a small matchbox)
- 2 to 3 ounces of beef, chicken, or fish (about the size of a deck of cards)

Portion distortion was observed almost thirty years ago. Researchers served people soup from a normal bowl to determine their normal intake, then on day four, they clandestinely substituted the normal bowls for bowls that were connected to hidden containers under the table. They slowly refilled the bowls as the participants ate. Both obese and lean participants ate more than their usual portions. **(1.23)** In another study volunteers were served increasingly larger portions of macaroni and cheese. This study also found that as the portion grew, so did the consumption. Each of these studies, as well as others, has found a consistent tendency in everyone to eat more when given a larger portion.

Dr. Barbara Rolls, one of the researchers in the mac-and-cheese study, determined, "Men and women, normal-weight and overweight individuals, restrained and unrestrained eaters, all responded to larger portion size by eating more." **(1.24)**

All Calories Are Not Equal

Calories alone will not help you get to your best health. If you eat 1,800 calories of snicker doodles, you are not going to feel or look as good as you could have had you eaten the proper balance of nutrients. Things just aren't that simple when it comes to the body. Sure, a calorie is a calorie whether it comes from a cookie or a carrot, but a calorie is really just a unit of measurement, like an inch or a pound. An inch is an inch whether you are measuring a nose or an ear. But there is a vast difference between a nose and an ear. Same goes with food—same unit of measurement, totally different purpose.

So what's the best ratio of carbohydrates, proteins, and fats? There's not really a one-size-fits-all as far as this is concerned. There is no magical percentage that will make the pounds disappear or add 20 years to your life. But finding a good ratio may help you feel better and allow you to reach your health goals. The amount of grams of carbohydrates, protein, and fat you should have depends on your body type and what you want to accomplish. For example, the optimal ratios for a thin male who wants to build muscle will be different than the ratios for an overweight female looking to lose weight.

Since most of us are not looking to enter the Mr. Universe contest or break a record for 26.1 miles, a good rule of thumb would be to use the recommendations by the Dietary Guidelines for Americans:

Carbohydrates: 45%–65%
Protein: 20%–35%
Fats: 10%–35% (less than 7% from saturated fats) (1.25)

Remember though that these ratios are not set in stone. They are just guidelines, and for the most part it is perfectly safe to make adjustments depending on your goals. For example, for weight loss, it's a good idea to decrease carbs and increase protein. A safe modification for weight loss would look something like this:

Carbohydrates: 40%
Protein: 35%
Fats: 25% (less than 7% from saturated fats)

I have a friend who is a professional bodybuilder. She goes as high as 40 to 50 percent protein. She keeps her healthy fats ratio high as well. Her ratio generally looks like this:

Carbohydrates: 30%
Protein: 45%
Fats: 25%

Marathon runners have a completely different set of needs. They need more carbs, so their ratios are lower in fats and proteins and can have carbohydrates up to 40 to 50 percent or more. **(1.26)**

In any case, it's a good idea to talk to your doctor to get a more specific plan tailored to your needs.

Simple Tips

There are also several apps and websites that will help you track your food, such as FitBit.com, MyFitnessPal.com, and MyFoodDiary.com. I do try and track what I eat in my FitBit account, but very rarely do I weigh my food out or try to get the numbers perfect. Most of the time I'm just living off general principles.

If you feel like your head is exploding with all of these ratios and numbers, take a deep breath. Unless you're planning on entering a body-building competition or competing in sports, you don't need to weigh every grape you put in your mouth. There are simple tricks to make balance easy.

1) PEACE PLATE RULE

One super simple technique to make sure you are getting the proper balance is to use something I call the Peace Plate Rule. The way this works is to take a 9-inch plate and draw an imaginary peace sign on it. One of the larger sections is for your non-starchy fruits and vegetables. The other large section is for protein. The two smaller sections are for your healthy grains/starches and healthy fats, or sometimes I'll use them for a healthy starch and a small dessert.

Remember that this only works on a 9-inch plate, and you may need to measure until you can recognize what that looks like. Just as portion sizes have increased, the average dinner plate has increased by 36 percent. Dinner plates have increased from 7 to 9 inches to 11 to 12 inches. Some restaurants use plates that are 13 inches across. No wonder we suffer from portion distortion!

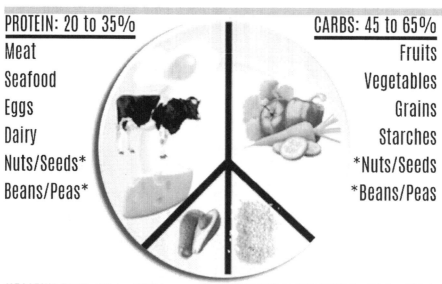

PROTEIN: 20 to 35%
Meat
Seafood
Eggs
Dairy
Nuts/Seeds*
Beans/Peas*

CARBS: 45 to 65%
Fruits
Vegetables
Grains
Starches
*Nuts/Seeds
*Beans/Peas

HEALTHY FATS: 10 to 35%
(less than 7% from Saturated)
Avocado
Olive Oil
Omegas
Nuts/Seeds

GRAINS & STARCHES: 10 to 15%
(or sometimes a treat)
Brown Rice
Quinoa
Sweet Potatoes
Whole Grains

2) PAIRING A CARB WITH A PROTEIN

Always try to pair a carborhydrate with a protein. Last week was my birthday. My daughter made me the best lemon cake on the planet. I decided that it was my special day, and I was going to enjoy. I enjoyed to the tune of one giant piece plus frosting. Then I had some Greek yogurt to balance it out. Sounds silly, but that added protein helped my blood sugar not go as crazy as it otherwise would have. Obviously most of the time I choose an apple or something healthier than a giant piece of birthday cake for my carb. **If you live healthy principles 85 to 90 percent of the time, you have some wiggle room to enjoy the yummy stuff without consequences.**

3) STEP AWAY FROM THE "NO-FAT" PRODUCTS

Obviously the no-fat diet phase was a complete bust. We need to get over our fear of fats, and if you opt for the 2 percent or whole milk instead of skim, you will have an automatic intake of fats. Don't be afraid of cheese and nuts and whipping cream, etc. Moderation is a better practice in this case than avoidance. Remember that you want about 25 percent of your diet to be healthy fats. Just stay away from those naughty trans fats.

4) THE SECRET WEAPON

Use healthy, pre-balanced meal replacements. When I ask my clients if they have heard eating every few hours is the healthiest way to do it, most of them say yes. My next question is always, "Is that what you are currently doing?"

Most of the time the answer to that is no. Generally it's because they are too busy or don't like preparing food or simply don't know what to eat. Healthy meal replacements are my #1 secret weapon to staying fit and getting in all of my nutrition. I don't leave home without them! One caveat, of course, is that you have to find a meal replacement that's actually healthy. Hint: If you're buying it at your regular grocery store, that's probably not the one you want. (If you would like a list of the products that I recommend, please visit my website, www.WendyHendry.com.).

Some folks are worried about the term "meal replacement." In my experience this is just a tool to help you accomplish your goals. Here's an example. One of my clients is also my lawn guy. When I suggested meal replacements, at first he didn't want to use "packaged food." I told him, "You know you could cut my grass with a pair of scissors, but it would be a lot easier to use your lawn mower." Again, healthy meal replacements are just a tool to help you accomplish your goals.

5) THE 3-BITE RULE FOR DESSERTS

I learned this helpful tip from one of my mentors, Dr. Wayne Scott Anderson. Anything more than three bites is waste for our taste buds. He writes in his book, "The first bite is the best tasting, the second not as good as the first and by the third, your taste bud experience is over so only take enough for 1 to 2 bites—just a taste and you will be surprised how satisfying it is." **(1.27)**

Trust the System

It's important to not limit yourself to certain foods while you're creating your new pattern of eating. If you find that eventually it's easier for you to not eat some specific trigger food, that's fine. But for right now, it's more important to just get used to eating on a regular schedule. Allow yourself to eat without beating yourself up. Also, don't worry too much about going over on your calories at this point. If anything, just make sure you don't go under. If you keep yourself undernourished or deprived, it's very difficult to reign in the urges. So figure out your caloric needs and then trust the system. I know it's scary. I've always been one that could never stop at one bite. It was all or nothing for me. While I was working on these physical health principles, I could stay deliberate for a few days or sometimes longer, but then I would "allow" myself a treat in order to not restrict, and I would end up bingeing.

If you find yourself in a similar situation, it's okay! Tell yourself that you're human and that everyone eats like that at times. How you talk to yourself becomes important in Section 2 where you will learn that be-rating yourself only weakens your willpower. So hang in there! The next section will get into the mental part of eating and how you can resist those urges to take more than a bite or two. But first you need to be feeding your body the right stuff and implementing a couple of other principles that will make being mindful much easier than it otherwise would.

> ## W.A.I.T.*loss* Challenge:
> Make sure you have some 9-inch plates and start now to follow the Peace Plate Rule. Try to choose healthy carbs, proteins, and fats most of the time, and follow the 3-Bite Rule for desserts.

Key #5: Exercise

What's more important, nutrition or exercise? The answer is both! In my case, exercise is what got me on the path to health. I could write an entire book on all of the different theories and opinions on how to exercise. Some say don't do cardio. Some say get in lots of cardio. Cardio makes you gain. Cardio makes you lose. Weight training is best. Cardio is good for your heart. Cardio is damaging to your heart, etc., etc., etc. After reading about a thousand different studies with a thousand different viewpoints, I decided to write and use references that are in line with my own personal experience.

When I first started Sweaty Chix Fitness™, I was a Tae Bo® addict. I would go down to California and train with Billy Blanks, Tae Bo® founder and kick-boxing king and was even able to be in some of his videos. When I first began exercising, I dropped my weight from 195 to about 150 pounds. During this time I really didn't focus as much on weight. I still binged at times, but I figured since I was so active, I didn't need to worry quite so much. Plus, the whole purpose of Sweaty Chix™ was to make women feel comfortable. Unfortunately, after a few years of daily cardio kick-boxing, I noticed that my pants were getting tighter around the waist (this was when I stepped on the scale to that surprising 170 pounds).

It made sense that I'd lost that 45 pounds at first, but I could not understand why, even with daily exercise, my weight went back up to 170

42

pounds. I had heard that to be fit, nutrition was 80 percent and exercise 20 percent. But I didn't think I was getting my 20 percent worth. Plus, my eating habits weren't perfect, but they were better than before I'd started exercising. Not only that, I realized that others in my classes were having the same problem. For as hard as we were working, we should have been getting smaller. Instead, we were getting bigger—and not in a good way.

I started researching, and here is what I learned: aerobic exercise is great for the newbie, but after a while, for some people, it becomes a "fat trap." If you're a cardio buff, don't hate me. I'm just stating the facts. Exercise is not an effective tool for losing weight. It's vital to overall health and weight maintenance, but if you're doing it simply to trim down, you may be disappointed with the outcome. There are several reasons for this scientific reality. **(1.28, 1.29)**

1) ADAPTIVE THERMOGENESIS

When we don't eat right, our body becomes protective of its resources and decreases our energy-making mechanisms to compensate for what it thinks may be lost. In other words, when I started exercising, I began burning more calories. When I began burning more calories, I lost weight. Because I lost weight and was still exercising and burning calories, my body thought it was starving, so it slowed down my metabolism. Since my calories and activity stayed the same, but my metabolism decreased, I began gaining weight again. No wonder I was so frustrated! The harder I worked to lose weight, the harder my body tried to resist losing weight. Was my body trying to sabotage my efforts? It does sort of seem that way, but in reality it's just our survival instinct kicking in to protect us from starving to death. Thank you, evolution!

Just be mindful of your body's ability to adapt to different conditions. If you notice yourself gaining weight, even though you're exercising regularly, re-evaluate your routine. You may need to adjust the type of exercise you're doing. **(1.30, 1.31)**

That brings us to the second body chemical saboteur.

2) CORTISOL AND OTHER HORMONES

Another way that our body undermines our efforts while protecting itself at the same time is by releasing a variety of hormones. One hormone that keeps us from losing weight during exercise is called cortisol. Cortisol is a hormone that is produced when we are exposed to a stressor. It helps wake up our fight-or-flight mechanism by dumping extra glucose into our muscles. Unfortunately, the body produces cortisol during intense exercise as well as when we are being chased by a bear.

People who are under chronic stress are especially susceptible to increased cortisol production and may find their exercise routines only exacerbate its effects. I've been to lots of cardio classes where the music is played loud enough to scare anyone. That along with an instructor yelling directions at us *should* alert our fight-or-flight to kick in! Generally, we exercise and then head to work or home where there is more stress and therefore, more cortisol. Chronic cortisol can cause a lot of problems, but it can specifically contribute to excess abdominal weight. Look around your aerobics class the next time you are there and see if the longtime students have an exercise belly like I did. **(1.32, 1.33, 1.34, 1.35)**

3) LESS CALORIES BURNED; MORE CALORIES CONSUMED

In the long run, cardio results in the loss of lean muscle mass. Lean muscle helps us burn more calories, which means the less of it we have, the less calories we burn. If our food intake doesn't change, we gain weight. This is a double downer as generally cardio increases the appetite, so our calorie intake actually increases.

Thankfully, there are some things that we can do to mitigate the negative effects of cardio activity. **(1.36, 1.37)**

• LIFT WEIGHTS. There is no ignoring the benefits of strength training. Resistance or strength training includes weight lifting as well as body weight exercises. And you don't need to train like Arnold Schwarzenegger to gain the benefits. Resistance training helps the metabolism stay revved up, and it also prevents muscle mass loss. **(1.38)**

• DON'T FORGET ABOUT THE PROTEIN. Remember that when we eat protein, our muscle mass is less likely to be depleted. Preserving muscle mass can help prevent adaptive thermogenesis that comes with weight loss and exercise. **(1.39)**

• TAKE A CHEAT DAY. Sometimes it's good to allow yourself to splurge a little. Studies show that this can help boost
the hormones that slow down energy expenditure. **(1.40)** A
cheat day doesn't mean that you stuff yourself until you're
sick. Be mindful, but allow yourself to enjoy some dessert or
a hamburger and fries.

So if exercise can lead to weight gain, why are we still doing it? Keep
in mind that by learning how to train properly, you can avoid any unwanted outcomes. But the fundamental reason to exercise is because the
benefits far outweigh the costs. Here are just a few:

1) IT'S THE ULTIMATE ANTI-DEPRESSANT!

If you want a brain boost every day, get up and move! As
we exercise, our body releases all sorts of feel-good hormones, including serotonin, dopamine, and norepineph-
rine. These are the happy hormones that boost mood and
keep us smiling. **(1.41)**

2) EXERCISING FOR 20 MINUTES LITERALLY MAKES OUR BRAINS BIGGER AND BETTER.

Studies have found that physical activity stimulates brain
cell growth and promotes a healthy environment for the
development of new neural pathways. In other words, it
helps with cognition and memory, and even strengthens willpower. In one study done by the Department of
Exercise Science at the University of Georgia, scientists
scanned the brains of participants who exercised for an
hour a day, three times a week for a period of six months.
They found that the part of the brain that controls mem-

ory and cognition actually grew in size. Apparently, when we work out, not only do we bulk up our muscles, we bulk up our brains! **(1.42, 1.43)**

3) EXERCISE PROMOTES A HEALTHY WEIGHT

Any unwanted calorie burned is a good thing, and exercise does indeed burn calories! Though there are reasons why it's not the best at helping us lose weight, it can definitely prevent weight gain and/or maintain weight loss.

4) EXERCISE BOOSTS OUR ENERGY

Regular physical activity strengthens our muscles and beefs up our endurance. When we move, oxygen and other nutrients are delivered to our muscles, and the cardiovascular system has to work harder. As our lungs and heart gain better endurance, we have more energy to get through the day.

5) EXERCISE CAN IMPROVE OUR SEX LIFE

There are studies that show exercise can lead to enhanced arousal for women and decreased erectile dysfunction for men. Enough said. **(1.44, 1.45)**

6) EXERCISE HELPS REDUCE EMOTIONAL EATING

Exercise reduces anxiety and stress, two of the most common triggers for grabbing comfort food.

7) EXERCISE CAN BE FUN!

Sometimes it takes trying a few different physical activities to find the one that is your perfect match. But it's out there somewhere, and once you find it, you will never be the same. It may be kick-boxing, weight lifting, yoga, racquetball, biking, running, or maybe even walking. Before you know it, you will be encouraging others to join you!

The 3 "Macro-Nutrients" of Exercise: Cardio, Strength, and Flexibility

I was so in love with cardio kick-boxing that I literally had to be forced out of my comfort zone into the unknown world of other formats, such as weights and yoga. I know now that stepping out of my little exercise bubble was the best thing I could have done. I knew well before doing the research that it takes a little bit of everything to see results. Kick-boxing gave me my endorphins and endurance, but weights and yoga gave me my sexy. It wasn't until combining all three exercise "macro-nutrients" that my arms, stomach, and everything else started firming up.

There have been years of studies over what kind of exercise is best: cardio vs. weight training vs. flexibility. The answer to that cliffhanger is that we need all three. Just like we need balance in our nutrition, we need balance in our physical activity. We can even apply the "Peace Plate Rule" to activity! It's okay to get a good dose of cardio and strength, but don't forget to add in some flexibility too. Oh, and for the dessert section of the plate, fill that up with FUN!

This type of cross training not only will help reduce cortisol, but it will reduce injury and produce the best possible results. **(1.46, 1.47)**

My Shout-Out to Yoga

Because I think it's the most well-rounded exercise, and it's one of the few exercises that reduces cortisol, I want to give a little extra plug for yoga. I only recently became a yoga addict. The first time I tried it was several years ago, and I must not have been in the right frame of mind. All I remember is peeking around during shavasana and thinking it was the weirdest thing I had ever done. I couldn't wait to get back to kick-boxing and loud music! Maybe it's because I'm older and have experienced teenagers and divorce, but now I relish the peace that comes with nostril breathing and Surya Namaskaras (sun salutations). I've found that the right yoga class can incorporate all three elements of exercise: cardio, strength, and flexibility. In other words, it's an all-inclusive workout! Additional benefits of incorporating yoga into your life include the following:

1) THERE ARE VERY FEW LIMITATIONS
You can easily modify to whatever level, age, and ability you are.

2) BETTER SLEEP
Yoga helps relax the nervous system so that not only is cortisol decreased, but also sleep comes easier and is more productive.

3) INCREASED STRENGTH

When you hold yoga positions, you will naturally strengthen your muscles. In this respect, yoga can also be considered body-weight resistance training.

4) DECREASED PAIN

The majority of the pain we feel is due to restricted motion and activity. Yoga helps decrease atrophy and helps us get moving in a gentle and smooth way. Also, as your alignment improves from the various poses, you will notice less pain as well as fewer injuries.

5) BETTER METABOLISM

Yoga increases your lean muscle and makes you more flexible. This alone is enough to get your metabolism going, but it also gives you more energy, making you more likely to be active throughout the day. **(1.48)**

6) BETTER BREATHING

It's important to focus on your breathing as you do yoga, and as you do so, you expand your lung capacity and can take deeper breaths. Breathing is as much a part of the practice as the positions and will improve right along with your headstands.

7) BETTER POSTURE AND BALANCE

Each pose performed in yoga is geared toward proper alignment and centering. The more you practice, the more you will find your posture and balance improving. The change may be gradual, but it will happen.

8) IMPROVED OVERALL HEALTH

Yoga has also been found to lower cholesterol, blood sugars, and heart disease. It helps decrease osteoporosis, improves memory, and boosts mood. **(1.49, 1.50, 1.51)**

W.A.I.T.*loss* Challenge:

If you have not been exercising regularly, start with the little things. Park a little farther away in the parking lots. Take the stairs instead of the elevator. Get up to change the channel on the television. If you are already exercising, mix things up. If you have been doing just cardio, take a pump class. Or if you hit the weights regularly, add in some cardio or flexibility.

Key #6: Water

Have you ever heard the story about the woman who always cut the end off of her ham before putting it in the roasting pan to bake? One time her daughter asked why she did that. Her mother replied, "Cause that's what *my* mom did." The daughter was curious and called grandma to ask why she cut the end off of the ham. Grandma replied that it was the only way the ham would fit into her roasting pan.

The point of this story is that sometimes we make up our own truths. I learned in doing research for this book that many of my ideas were really just "cutting off the end of the ham." In other words, I've been teaching "truths" with no scientific backup. Water consumption was the one that surprised me the most.

I've preached for years the value of drinking, at the minimum, 64 ounces of water a day. When I sat down to write this chapter, I thought it would be the easiest one of all to prove. I thought I'd read and cite a few studies that show why we need to drink at least eight 8-ounce glasses of water a day, and I would move on to the next chapter. That did not prove to be the case.

As I read through dozens of clinical studies on water, I could not find any solid scientific evidence showing that we are doomed if we do not get in a certain amount.

One Oxford study concluded the following:

This study does not support the recommendation that people should consume at least eight glasses of fluid each day. More and better evidence is needed before encouraged fluid or water intake is known to be both beneficial and safe. Until then, we suggest specific fluid intake targets are not appropriate in general health advisory statements. Similarly, specific water intake advisories are not warranted based on the lack of currently available evidence. **(1.52)**

The Institute of Medicine, an agency that advises the Federal Government, says that most healthy people can simply let thirst be their guide. It does not specify exact requirements for water. **(1.53)**

I feel almost scandalous debunking the 64-ounce minimum myth, and I want to make something absolutely clear. I *still* endorse drinking lots of water every day, but the bottom line is all of these minimum recommendations that we hear about are subjective. There is no scientific endorsement as to how much we should be drinking.

Now that we've cleared that up, I want to spend the rest of the chapter telling you why it's still important in water's case to "cut off the end of the ham" and drink up! First of all, we need water to survive. Our body is made of about 60 percent water. Our brain is 70 percent water, and our lungs weigh in at almost 90 percent water. We lose about 3 to 4 cups of water every day through urine, sweat, and other body excretions. We lose 1 to 2 liters just by breathing!

Even though the 64-ounce a day rule has not been substantiated, it's better to err on the side of too much water than too little. A good rule of thumb is to drink half your body weight in ounces. So if you weigh 150 pounds, shoot for 75 ounces of water.

Here are some fact-checked reasons to drink up:

1) WATER HELPS IN WEIGHT LOSS

One very good reason to keep on drinking is that water does play a part in increased weight loss. One study showed that over a 12-week time period, those who drank 2 cups of water before a meal lost over 5 pounds more than those who didn't. In similar fashion, another study showed that drinking water could cause mild increases in metabolism. It's estimated that drinking 2 liters (68 ounces) in one day can burn about 96 calories. **(1.54, 1.55)**

2) WATER KEEPS YOUR DIGESTION MOVING ALONG

This is not something you want to talk about at the dinner table, but if you don't drink enough water, the colon pulls it from the stools. That increases your risk of constipation and makes things generally more uncomfortable. Water also helps flush out toxins, therefore, relieving some of the burden on the kidneys.

3) WATER HELPS FIGHT WORK-OUT FATIGUE

A lot of water is lost when we exercise. Not only does replacing that prevent dehydration, but maintaining fluid balance can improve endurance and prevent exhaustion. Remember also that water is just as important during cold-weather workouts as summer sweat fests. Cold weather can weaken thirst as we lose fluid through respiration as well as sweating through extra layers of clothing.

4) WATER HELPS THE BRAIN WORK

Dehydration actually causes brain cells to shrink. Being dehydrated by just 2 percent impairs functions that require attention and certain memory skills. So when we are water deficient, our brains have to work a lot harder. One study showed that students who enter the exam halls with a water bottle actually perform better on tests. **(1.56, 1.57)**

5) WATER MAY HELP YOU LIVE LONGER

Water may actually keep you from dying of heart disease. Research has shown that increased water consumption can reduce the risk of death from coronary heart disease. **(1.58)**

6) WATER CAN GIVE YOU A BETTER ATTITUDE

Drinking water can help improve your mood! Increased daily water intake has been shown to lighten the disposition of those who normally drink lower amounts of water. The opposite has also been shown; those who usually drink lots of water have a negative shift in mood when intake decreases. Even mild dehydration can bring you down. **(1.59)**

7) WATER MAY HELP PREVENT HEADACHES, NATURALLY

One of my daughters suffers from migraines. I always knew it was linked to food as her migraines always come on if she hasn't eaten in a while. But after reading several studies, I'm wondering if it's a lack of water that is to blame. In one study, 50 migraine sufferers were asked if they believed insufficient fluid intake could have provoked their migraine attacks. Over half replied positively. Many headache sufferers have also experienced "total relief" within 30 minutes of drinking an average of 2 cups of water. **(1.60, 1.62)**

These benefits are all wonderful, but one of the biggest reasons that I am rarely seen without a water bottle in my hand is because it's a great reminder to W.A.I.T. before sticking something else, such as a cake pop, into my mouth. In the next section, we are going to talk about Habit Loops and how it's possible to replace one habit action with another. In some ways, drinking water has served this purpose for me.

W.A.I.T *loss* Challenge:
For one solid week, have a water bottle within reach and use it as a reminder to W.A.I.T.

Bonus Challenge:

Drink a couple of glasses of water before a meal and see if you don't start consuming fewer calories. Science says it works. (1.63)

Section 2: W.A.I.T.
Mindful Health

When Frank McNally wrote the *History of Ireland in 100 Excuses,* the fifth excuse was "The Spirit is willing, but the flesh is weak." I'm sure that particular biblical idiom can explain away a lot of bygones and not just the Irish ones! **(2.1)**

All of us have experienced the frustration of our body and our mind wanting separate things. My hope for you in this section is that you learn that you are not as weak as you think you are. As a matter of fact, your "flesh" is all in your head, literally, and there is no craving that you cannot conquer.

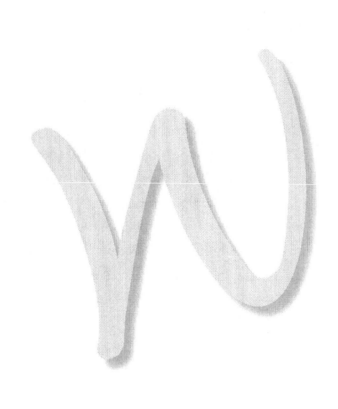

Wendy's Story

Wendy's Story

Dysfunctional to Functional

I was never asked to a dance while I was in high school. The only reason I was able to go to my senior prom was because I asked one of the high school students that I tutored to take me. It was not the romantic evening I had dreamed of. He was great, but I had to drive my mom's Pinto. That kind of says it all right there. Looking back, I'm glad I spent most of my high school as a big girl. I think my lack of self-confidence kept me from getting into trouble, and I know it forced me to develop a personality.

By the time I went to college, I was desperate for a boyfriend. Food could keep me company in the evenings and on weekends, but it couldn't hold my hand and make me feel cool on campus. I dieted hard the summer before college to lose weight, and by the time September rolled around, I was thin again. I was starting a whole new life in college and was determined that everyone would know me as the thin and happy girl.

The new me paid off in the form of a boyfriend named Bob. Bob was one of the nicest guys I had ever met. He liked to take me shopping for all sorts of things, especially clothes. At the beginning of the year they were size small, but by Christmas, I was sporting a large again. The bingeing had started the second week of school. I was so disgusted with myself. Poor Bob. All of a sudden I went from this fun, cute "new" Wendy to the depressed, bloated "old" Wendy who could barely force herself out of bed. I put on 40 pounds and was miserable.

I could not understand why I couldn't eat like a normal person. My roommates were all "normal" people. They could eat half of a candy bar and save the rest for later. They could have ice cream in the fridge until it went bad (or until I ate it without them knowing). They could go on a date and not think about food the entire time. For me, one bite always turned into a face-stuffing free-for-all, and excursions ended early so I could come home and binge. It became a routine to come home from school and eat until I was sick. I think the only reason I didn't gain more than 40 pounds was because I would starve myself after bingeing. Sometimes I could go two days without eating. It became a complete all-or-nothing. I was either starving myself, or I was stuffing myself. The crazy thing is that no matter how many times this went on, every time I finished a binge, I would swear it was the last one.

When I was 21, I went to live in Argentina for 18 months. I was there as a missionary for my church. I wish I could say that my binge-ing didn't affect my service, but it did. You can't *not* eat in Argentina. Their food is amazing! Dulce de leche ice cream, noquis, alfajores, bread. I started my mission at about 150 pounds. By the end of the first 8 months, I was 80 kilos. (Argentina uses the metric system. That's 175 pounds. To this day, I count my blessings that I got parasites right before I came home and walked off the plane a cool 140 pounds.) Even on my mission I wondered why others didn't seem as obsessed as I was about food. I lived to wake up and eat breakfast, and I looked forward all day to the next meal. The other missionaries could walk right past the heladeria (ice cream shop) without rubbernecking.

After Argentina, I finished school, got married, had kids, got divorced, got re-married, had more kids. I worked in laboratories, hospitals, and owned my own businesses. In other words, my life carried on and my situations changed, but my eating habits did not. I went to various therapists and even tried hypnotism, but I could not get a grip on my bingeing. Sometimes it consumed me to the point where I thought it would be easier to just be dead.

Between the time my doctor told me to lose 20 pounds and the day my mom had her stroke, my friend recommended a program that she had used to help her get healthy and lose weight. She said she could teach me the things she learned and that it would help me lose weight. I was very skeptical. She was very persistent. After I gave her several brush-offs and some snarky remarks, I finally relented. I learned all of the habits and principles I have shared in this book, and I did indeed lose weight. As a matter of fact, after implementing all of these Keys, I ended up at about 125 pounds. I hadn't weighed 125 since my high school experience with Dana. I was still skeptical about keeping the weight off long term, but the months flew by, and my weight stayed put, give or take 10 pounds depending on my binge frequency.

Even more important than helping me lose weight, I learned about eating every few hours, balancing my meals, drinking my water, and the other healthy Keys to help me to break free from a lifetime of "diet mentality." Since I was eating some protein every few hours, I didn't have hunger to trigger me, but even better, I quit restricting. My binge frequency decreased, and when I did binge, I would immediately get right back on track living these Key Principles of good health. I was really surprised that even though I was still bingeing at times, I could, for the most part, maintain my weight without restriction. I felt like half the battle had been won.

I decided at that point to become a health coach so I could tell the whole world about how easy it is to get healthy. I knew the first time I saw one of my clients experience true health that I had found my life's work. The only problem was I still couldn't seem to control my sporadic binge eating, and at times I felt like a huge hypocrite. Here I was, claiming to be a professional health coach, yet I could easily put away three bowls of ice cream and a box of sugar cereal an hour before bedtime. Why couldn't I say no to my cravings? My obsessive desire to figure that out was fueled by the fact that many of my clients had the exact same issue. I wanted to help them as much or more than I wanted to help myself.

I had been a coach for about a year when help came in the form of a book called *Brain over Binge: Why I Was Bulimic, Why Conventional Therapy Didn't Work, and How I Recovered for Good*. *Brain over Binge* is the personal story of Kathryn Hansen and her seven-year struggle with bulimia (and yes, this is the wonderful author who wrote the Foreword for this book!). The second I started reading her book I knew it was going to help me. It wasn't like any binge book I had ever read or any advice I had ever been given by a counselor. Traditionally, food disorder and eating addiction treatments have been based on coping with veiled emotional problems. Most therapists, including mine, taught that you have to address the emotional reasons behind the addiction before you can fix the addiction. I'd been trying to fix my crazy for 35 years.

In *Brain over Binge*, Kathryn shares an experience she had while taking a medication usually prescribed for migraines. While she was taking the medicine, her bingeing stopped. It wasn't her emotions that had changed or her dysfunctional childhood experiences. The only difference was that her urges had disappeared. She came to understand that if she could rid herself of her urges, she could rid herself of her bingeing. Eventually she learned that the power to do just that lay within her own mind.

Brain over Binge was the first time I had ever heard that I might actually have the power within myself to quit bingeing. For years I thought stopping a binge through willpower alone was as impossible as stopping my heart. I thought I was a victim of addiction "disease." For years I had prayed for God to take away this awful affliction when in reality, I had the choice to quit all along.

Kathryn learned how to recognize her urges for what they actually were—a "childish" part of her brain just trying to get its way. By using the more "adult" part of her brain, she learned to control her cravings and eventually make them disappear. In *Brain over Binge*, Kathryn wrote:

> What if I could separate myself from my urges and choose not to follow them anymore? *Perhaps,* I thought, *in spite of even the most powerful urge, I could choose not to open the refrigerator, not to drive to the convenience store; and maybe if I did that over and over, the urges would simply go away on their own.* I decided to try what I'd learned. **(2.2)**

Through this self-awareness Kathryn was able to stop bingeing immediately. I learned so much reading her book, but unfortunately, it wasn't as easy for me to quit. I still had a lot to learn. But I am so grateful to *Brain over Binge* as it became the first step on my path to recovery and opened up a whole new world of self-awareness to me.

Our Amazing Brain

Have you ever noticed that you have two voices in your head? For example, when you see a crème filled donut and you smell that sugary goodness, Voice #1 commands, *"Eat the donut!"* while Voice #2 advises, *"Step away from the donut!"* We hear two voices because different parts of our brains have different purposes, and at times they act like a checks-and-balances system.

The Limbic System (aka The Bratty Brain)

Voice #1, the one goading us to eat the donut, originates from a part of the brain that begins developing at birth called the limbic system. The limbic system is buried deep inside the cerebrum and is responsible for feelings and emotions as well as self-preservation and survival. It is also involved in behavior motivation and reinforcement. In other words, it wants us to be gratified and feel pleasure. It's impulsive and impetuous and sometimes a little reckless, but it's not the enemy. I used to picture the limbic system as the little devil on my shoulder, but then I learned that even though at times it seduces me to do things I regret, it is also responsible for keeping me alive. **(2.3)**

This part of our brain is very primitive, both biologically and evolutionarily speaking, and is, for the most part, something we have in common with many primitive animals. The animal limbic system plays an important role in defending territory, hunting, and eating prey— the survival stuff. When an animal is hungry, it doesn't stop to analyze whether or not eating is going to make it fat. It just eats. **(2.4)**

The purpose of the limbic system in humans is basically the same, to make us do things on instinct so that we survive. When a bear is chasing us, there is no time to stop and think. We have to react! Because the limbic system is responsible for keeping us alive, it needs a way to get our attention fast! That's why the urges and cravings that we feel are so powerful. When we drive past the Krispy Kreme® and the urge tells us to make a U-turn, it's really just our limbic system "yelling" for food.

The limbic system is composed of several small sections of the brain which scientists decided to lump together as the "limbic system" in the 1940s. It's been called many different things including: animal brain, spoiled child, beast brain, primitive brain, and emotion center. Freud called it the Id. Because it annoys me and sometimes won't shut up, I call it my "bratty brain" or "The Brat." The limbic system is one of the first parts of our brain to develop and is fully functional before our second birthday. It's this impulsive part of our Brat brain that pretty much controls us until we are in our early twenties. (If you have raised teenagers, this explains a lot.)

The Pre-Frontal Cortex (aka PFC)

Voice #2 is the one prompting us to put the donut back in the box. It's called the pre-frontal cortex and is responsible for our cognition or thought processes. The pre-frontal cortex also has several descriptive nicknames including thinking brain, objectionable observer, gatekeeper, and the boss. This part of the brain is what Freud referred to as the Ego.

Unlike animals, the reason we can pause before eating is because we have the ability to reason. Our PFC gives us the power to use logic and to contemplate. Without our PFC, we couldn't plan, solve problems, learn from past experiences.

The PFC looks out for our best interests and encourages us to choose wisely. When The Brat, the one that wants immediate pleasure, tries to convince me to smoke a cigarette, it's my PFC that reminds me that it's not worth dying of lung cancer. When The Brat sees an expensive pair of stilettos and urges me to spend more money than I should, it's my PFC that talks me out of it. (If they are really sexy, sometimes The Brat wins that one.) When The Brat smells something yummy, it beckons me to indulge. Anyway, you get the point. In each of these situations, it is the pre-frontal cortex, PFC, that considers my best interests and then makes the choice.

The Two-Part Brain Theory

Jack Trimpey, a licensed clinical social worker, began to challenge the addiction "disease" philosophy supported by Twelve-Step programs when he realized his own urges for alcohol were coming from his limbic system. He founded an approach called the Addictive Voice Recognition Technique (AVRT), which gives "voice" to the destructive urges coming from The Brat. The principle behind AVRT is to use mindfulness to separate your "two voices" and to recognize that for the addict, The Brat's sole purpose is to feel good and to consume. According to Trimpey, The Brat is not really you at all but is actually your strongest opponent. It's just a voice in your head wanting to get high and feel pleasure. On the other hand, the pre-frontal cortex is who you really are. *You* are the sensible one, and *you* want what is in your best interest. It's just that The Brat is relentless in wanting what it wants. **(2.5)**

I like how Trimpey explains it:

Your [pre-frontal cortex] . . . is not only many times larger than your mid-brain, but is also the most sophisticated organization of matter in the known universe. It can master both its physical and psychological environments. Given the correct information, the human [pre-frontal cortex] (yes, you) is able to suppress any appetite, able to defeat any addiction, any time you choose. **(2.6)**

In other words, you can unmask The Brat's true colors, and then you can destroy it!

Though it's written specifically for substance abuse, Trimpey's book *Rational Recovery: The New Cure for Substance Addiction* is how Kathryn Hansen learned that she had the power inside her own mind to not binge. She learned to disassociate herself (the PFC) from the urges coming from The Brat. In other words, she heard them but didn't react. She just observed them without emotion, as if they weren't coming from her at all. She acknowledged them and then chose not to comply. Eventually The Brat voice prompting her to binge got quieter and quieter until after a while, it was gone. **(2.7)**

I'm embarrassed to admit this, but until I read *Brain over Binge*, I had no idea what it meant to be mindful. I tried to understand it. I pretended to understand it. At times I even thought I did understand it, but I was way off.

Everything I read about mindfulness sounded like some new age guru practice. Definitions included words like *self-awareness, present moment, space of freedom, state of being conscious*, etc. All of these terms were out of the scope of my understanding. I look back now and realize that the reason I didn't understand was because I was about as far away from being mindful as anyone possibly could be. One time I had a friend tell me that she couldn't be around me for very long because I was frenetic. I took it as a compliment until I looked up the definition of frenetic. It means frantic and crazy! Basically, it's the opposite of peaceful and calm. Although I do think a better adjective for me is distracted, I didn't want to be frantic OR distracted. I just didn't know how to be anything else. My mind was always on high speed, and most of the time it was focused on anything but what it should be.

Brain over Binge turned the light on for me. Once I understood that I had two competing voices and that the binges were just my survival instincts throwing a temper tantrum, I started to understand what it meant to be mindful. Mindfulness is *self*-awareness, or separating "The Self" from "The Brat."

In one part of her book, Kathryn recommends that the reader sit down and really listen to the limbic system and the pre-frontal cortex "speak" to each other. I still remember the first time I did that. I sat down in my living room where it was quiet, and I just focused. It took some mental effort, but eventually the voices emerged like a hologram. It was like I was eavesdropping on my own thoughts. I had never consciously "heard" them before, and it was a completely new experience for me. Kathryn was able to stop bingeing right away, and some of my clients have experienced the same immediate results. It wasn't as easy for me. I didn't stop bingeing right away though I did begin to hear my addictive voice. Sometimes I was able to ignore it, and sometimes I wasn't. My binges did become less frequent, and when I did succumb to the urges, I was more cognizant of my poor choice.

Though I wasn't cured, I did have more hope than I ever had. The *Brain over Binge* principles did work for me, and even if it was intermittent, it was real. I knew if I could just strengthen my PFC, I could conquer The Brat once and for all. I just needed to know how to strengthen my ability to walk away. I needed to somehow beef up my willpower.

> **W.A.I.T.*loss* Challenge:**
> The next time you feel a craving coming on, go to a quiet place and just try to "hear" your thoughts. See if you can follow the steps that Kathryn used to quit bingeing. First, separate yourself from the urge and acknowledge it like a bystander. Second, make the conscious choice to ignore it.

Key #7: Brain Exercise

In the beginning of Section 2, we talked about our pre-frontal cortex (PFC) being the part of our brain that looks out for our best interest. It makes sense then that our willpower and self-regulation are housed in this section of our mind.

In my research on the subject, I found a book called *Willpower: Rediscovering the Greatest Human Strength* by Dr. Roy Baumeister, a professor at Florida State University. He has become one of the leading experts on willpower and self-regulation, and has shown in study after study that willpower actually functions much like a muscle, even to the extent that it is a limited resource.

Decision Fatigue

Not only can willpower be strengthened like a muscle, it can also be worn out and depleted. In one of Baumeister's studies, participants who used their willpower to resist chocolate were afterwards less able to continue doing a difficult self-control exercise. Another experiment forced participants to remain unemotional during a sad movie. Subsequently, they also more quickly abandoned the exercises requiring self-control. These studies showed that even simple daily tasks used up our willpower energy and that we have a limited supply of self-control. Dr. Baumeister coined this new insight "decision fatigue." **(2.8, 2.9)**

Decision fatigue, or willpower depletion, explains, among other things, why we have the afternoon and evening munchies. From the minute we get up in the morning until the time we go to bed, we are making decisions and carrying out tasks that drain our PFC. In the morning, our willpower is rested and strong. By the time lunch rolls around it's exhausted and ready for a break. Do you, like most people, find it a lot harder to resist temptation in the afternoon than in the morning? When our willpower is exhausted, we are at the mercy of The Brat.

Decision fatigue affects more than just appetite. It affects everything we do. One study examined over 1,000 parole board rulings. The purpose of the rulings was to determine whether or not to release the criminal from prison. The researchers found that instead of basing their decisions on the type of crime committed, the parole judges' decisions were more about the time of day. Prisoners who appeared first thing in the morning received parole about 70 percent of the time. Those who appeared later in the day received a less than 10 percent chance of a favorable ruling. **(2.10)**

Willpower Conditioning

Some people are born with amazing muscle tone. It is a gift they just have from birth and developing defined muscles is easy for them. Neither muscle strength nor definition comes naturally to me. I have to work for it every day. Our PFC acts under the same principle. Some people are born with stronger willpower "muscle" tone than others. Obviously, my willpower, like my biceps, was a little wimpy and needed some heavy lifting.

The point of brain exercise is the same as body exercise, to consistently get endurance and competence. So every time you resist an urge, it's like lifting a mental barbell. In short, self-control begets self-control.

Take note that you don't want to fight against the urge anymore than you want to kick a heavy weight. That's counterproductive. You want to acknowledge it, respect it, and then firmly use your PFC to ignore it.

Understanding Mental Exercises

It's really important that you understand how the brain works because the addicted bratty part of our brain wants us to think in all-or-nothing terms. In my other attempts at using willpower to not binge, it was a battle. It was me against "The Binge." So when the "The Binge" finally won the battle, which it eventually always did, I would think to myself, "I knew you couldn't keep this up! I knew you would give in!" Well, of course I was going to give in! The mental resistance as well as the negative self-talk was using up my willpower energy so that eventually it was bound to fatigue. Plus, instead of finding a new routine, I was just gritting my teeth to make it through. It felt like I was walking around carrying a thousand pounds on my back. Eventually I was going to crumble, and when I did, I was so internally exhausted that I gave up. I figured that was it. I was never going to be able to get better. Might as well eat a few dozen cookies and a pizza.

Understanding that our willpower can strengthen with each good choice means that one binge doesn't mess up everything. You don't need to worry about the "one" binge; instead, focus on the one time you ignored it. If you have three urges to binge in a day, and you resist just one of them, it's like you lifted a ten-pound weight, so the next day you will be a little stronger and able to resist *two* urges. There is no carrying around a thousand pounds. There is no wasting energy on negativity because with each resisted urge, you've mentally exercised your willpower and strengthened it a little more for the next time.

It took me several months before my urges began to disappear. I would resist one and then choose to not resist the next one. Then I would resist two, then back to one, then three, etc. Meanwhile, the time between urges began to spread out and weaken because my willpower muscle was getting stronger. I rarely get the urge to binge anymore, and when I do, I have control over my choice.

So if you don't stop bingeing right away, it's okay. Could you walk into the gym and start squatting with 200 pounds on your back? Look at the incremental growth instead of feeling sorry for yourself because you aren't ripped after one visit to the gym. Willpower exercise is no different. With each good decision, you are getting stronger, and your ability to mentally lift more "weight" is growing. Celebrate what you *have* accomplished, not what you haven't!

Brain Fueling

We talked in Section 1 about proper fueling for the body. Proper fueling is also imperative for the mind. Decision-making is not the only thing affected by a lack of fuel. Willpower, ability to reason, use of logic, and all cognitive skills become depleted when the PFC is low on energy. **(2.11)**

Just like our muscles, the brain is a bit of a sugar junkie. It can use fat for fuel if it needs to, but it much prefers glucose. Understanding the role of glucose in the brain answers a lot of questions. The brain is only about 2 percent of our body weight, but it uses about 33 percent of the calories we consume. When blood sugar drops, one of the first symptoms is confusion and brain fog. Have you ever noticed that if you go too long without food it's harder to concentrate and focus?

The importance of glucose also explains a lot of our cravings. I always know when my period is about to roll around because I would cut off my arm or bite off someone's head to have chocolate. Since our PFC is not necessary for our survival, it is the first thing to give up energy (glucose) when another part of the body calls. Therefore, willpower is drained whenever we are sick or have an injury because extra glucose is needed for immunity and healing. When we are pregnant or having our period, our PFC gives up some of its fuel to help with those things. Same goes with stress and anger and other emotions. All of these things drain our PFC, which means our willpower is weaker and The Brat's voice is louder, bossier, and more demanding. **(2.12, 2.13, 2.14, 2.15)**

The discoveries about glucose help explain why dieting is a particularly difficult test of self-control—and why even people with normally strong willpower can have such a hard time losing weight. We start out the day with virtuous intentions, resisting croissants at breakfast and dessert at lunch, but each act of resistance further lowers our willpower. As our willpower weakens late in the day, we need to replenish it. But to resupply that energy, we need to give the body glucose. In other words, we're trapped in a nutritional catch-22: in order not to eat, a dieter needs willpower, but in order to have willpower, a dieter needs to eat. **(2.16)**

The keys to gaining a healthy mind then are the same keys used to gain a healthy body. You start by eating the right foods in the right balance. Choosing your carbs from the low glycemic list, balancing those with your protein and fat, and of course doing mental exercise.

Key #8: Quiet Time/ Meditation

One thing that I've always found a little ironic in weight lifting is if you overwork a muscle group, it's counterproductive. Muscles need time to rest and rejuvenate. This principle also applies to our thinking brain. I mentioned previously that willpower is not an unlimited resource, but neither is decision fatigue a permanent condition. Just like a cell phone battery, the PFC, including willpower, can be recharged. Obviously a good night's sleep will recharge your willpower battery, but you can also do a quick revive anytime. As a bonus, while your brain is recharging, it's also upgrading. That is to say, the same method used to renew your depleted PFC can strengthen it at the same time. The training method is called meditation.

Just as with my naive concept in regards to mindfulness, I thought meditation was for Buddhists and people that like yoga. To me, meditation meant sitting cross-legged with my thumb and finger touching together like a teardrop in the air. In my mind quiet time and meditation were two separate things. Quiet time meant taking a two-hour nap. And though I did teach my clients to have "quiet time," I never realized that it could actually solve the afternoon munchies dilemma. Even though I always woke up from a nap more drowsy than before, I thought a two-hour afternoon nap counted as quiet time. I don't know why it didn't dawn on me that maybe that type of quiet time wasn't a "healthy habit" after all

Once I became educated about the subject, I came to realize that meditation and quiet time are a team and together can be a very effective "battery-recharging" tool. It only takes a few minutes of meditation during quiet time for our thinking brain "battery" to be back up to 100 percent power.

Just as there are many different fitness exercises to train and strengthen the body, there are many meditation exercises that can be used to build up and challenge the mind. **(2.17)**

One of the easiest ways to start meditating is by focusing on a single point and then refocusing every time the mind wanders from that point. This technique is called concentration meditation and can be as simple as focusing on our breathing.

The first time I tried, it was pure torture for me. I lay on my bed with my feet up and put one hand on my heart and one on my stomach. I started taking deep breaths in my nose and out my mouth. By the time I had finished the second breath, my brain had moved on to some other topic . . . probably what I was going to eat for dinner. As soon as I found my mind wandering, I began focusing on my breathing again . . . Breathe in, breathe out, breath in, breathe . . . *Where did Chloe say she was going after school? I wonder if she fed the dog before she left? I think I can hear the dog chewing on something in the bathroom . . . I forgot to turn off my curling iron . . . When is my hair appointment again? Ugh. Too many distractions! Focus.* Breathe in, breathe out, breathe . . . *I need to remember to put so-and-so's birthday on my calendar . . . Did I remember to call so-and-so? . . . Why is my house so quiet? Where are the kids? . . .* Anyway, you get my drift. I couldn't focus for even two minutes. I'm sorry to say that this first foray into concentration meditation was not a success. I finally got up, frustrated, and crossed it off my to-do list.

The next time I decided to give meditation a try again was after attending a presentation by Dr. Gordon Bruin, a professional counselor who specializes in the education and treatment of addiction issues. In his book, *The Language of Recovery,* Dr. Bruin outlines the meditation technique that he teaches to his struggling clients:

> To begin the process, I invite you to memorize a meaningful [passage] or a favorite positive quote, something uplifting and encouraging. Once the passage is memorized, you are ready to begin the meditation process. When meditating, it is recommended that you find a quiet place so you can be undisturbed. Find a place to be comfortable, sitting in a chair with your feet and arms resting comfortably. At the outset, choose a specific amount of time you will be meditating. It is suggested you begin with five minutes. This will increase in time, but start slowly as you begin. Five minutes may seem like an eternity when you are not accustomed to doing this. This form of proactive meditation is quite simple. Close your eyes, relax and then begin by repeating the words of your memorized passage. For the next five minutes, do nothing but slowly and deliberately repeat the words of your chosen passage over and over again. As you do so, pay close attention to what is going on in your mind. You will quickly begin to notice the multitude of thoughts that will begin distracting you. The purpose of this form of meditation is to simply notice those distractions and then gently bring your

mind back to the task of repeating the verse or passage. This is a simple but powerful practice that can strengthen the [thinking brain's] ability to become more aware of what is happening in the mind from moment to moment.

I picked a short verse and decided to give Dr. Bruin's method a shot. I think my previous attempt at self-awareness actually prepared me to try again because my expectations were much less than the actual experience. That's not to say my mind didn't wander from my chosen passage, but I was more able to refocus this time. My goal had been to meditate for five minutes. I was surprised that when I was done, fifteen minutes had passed. I don't think I'll ever be able to meditate for hours on end like many Buddhists practice, but I can go a good thirty minutes now, and I am able to bring my mind back much more easily now. The real trick is to not let the peacefulness put you to sleep!

One important fact: you can't do sit-ups for a few days and expect a six-pack. In the same respect, you have to give self-awareness exercises time to do their job. Despite my first negative experience with meditation, something that Dr. Bruin said helped me understand this wisdom:

I have some clients that have disciplined themselves to do this meditation for 30 to 40 minutes per session. The benefits of consistently doing it are remarkable, but you have to keep doing it on a consistent basis.

Pumping mental "weights" or practicing these exercises can literally build up your brain bulk. A study done a few years ago at Harvard found that after eight weeks of daily, 30-minute meditation, study participants actually increased the gray-matter density in the areas of the brain associated with self-awareness and deep thought. In other words, their brains grew bigger! **(2.18, 2.19)**

The unfortunate thing for me is that unless I meditate on the toilet, I generally don't have 30 uninterrupted minutes in a day. Luckily, just like a cell phone, you don't need a 100 percent battery to be able to get through the day. You just need enough to get it turned on and running. I've found that even a small break during the day extends my "battery" life. The researchers that conducted the study on the inadvertent parole board decisions found that after the judges took a lunch break, each prisoner's odds of a favorable ruling jumped back up. On busy days, even a few minutes of deep breathing can work wonders.

Along with giving us the mind power to resist our impulsive urges, meditation has been shown to decrease blood pressure, improve breathing, decrease stress, and strengthen the immune system. There are many other medical benefits that researchers are just now discovering.

W.A.I.T.*loss* Challenge:
Find a quiet place and practice some form of concentration meditation. Start with five minutes and set a goal to focus for 15 to 30 minutes each day.

Key #9: Sleep

I always gained more weight after having a baby than during the pregnancy. I remember once someone asking me when the baby was due. The "baby" was two at the time. I attribute my after-baby weight gain to my after-baby lack of sleep. I did eat at night sometimes because I needed the energy to stay awake, but the calories consumed at 3 am did not equate to the 40 to 60 pounds gained over the year following birth.

College was another period of my life where I rarely got more than 5 or 6 hours of sleep. I remember staying up all night in college and polishing off a pizza and a quart of ice cream all by myself. I have several clients that work graveyard shifts and report munching all night long. I remember my dad delivering the *LA Times* out of our van. He would get up at 3 am and finish up around 6 am. He always came home with a half-eaten box of donuts.

There are literally hundreds of studies that show the relationship between sleep deprivation and weight gain, and I'm betting that most of us have our own stories to back up the correlation. Sleep deprivation and food go hand in hand.

People who don't get enough sleep consume an average of 300 calories more than their well-rested counterparts. They also snack more and exercise less. That would make sense if they ate only enough to cover the calories burned to keep them awake, but they actually eat much more than is needed.

A study done at the University of Colorado monitored 16 young, lean, healthy adults. The participants had to live for 2 weeks at the University of Colorado Hospital and were able to sleep for 9 hours the first 3 nights. After baseline measurements were established, the group was split into two. One group spent 5 days being able to get only 5 hours of sleep each night. The other lucky group was able to get in 9 hours. Both groups were fed big meals and were able to snack throughout the day. The snack options ranged from fruit and yogurt to ice cream and chips. After the first 5-day period the groups switched. On average, those who slept 5 hours a night burned 5 percent more energy than those who slept 9 hours a night, but they ate 6 percent more calories. Those with less sleep also tended to eat less in the morning and then binge after dinner. The research also showed that the participants who didn't get enough sleep consumed more carbohydrates and gained nearly 2 pounds in that short period of time. **(2.20, 2.21)**

We can also blame two hormones, ghrelin and leptin, for causing sleep-related weight gain. Ghrelin is produced in the stomach and sends messages to the LS telling it to increase hunger. Leptin does the opposite. It is produced by fat cells and tells the LS to decrease hunger when there's an excess of storage. Simply stated, ghrelin is the "I'm hungry" signal, and leptin is the "I'm full" signal. **(2.22)**

Lack of sleep boosts ghrelin production and diminishes leptin production. In other words, sleep deprivation imitates starvation so that we eat even when our energy stores don't need replenishing. Researchers have also found that regular sleep patterns (especially regular wake times) were most strongly linked with lower body fat. **(2.23)**

It's important that we listen to our internal clocks. Not heeding our biological warnings can cause weight gain, but it also increases risk of heart disease and failure, high blood pressure, stroke, diabetes, and slower cognition.

I've included the National Sleep Foundation's recommended amount of sleep, but generally speaking, if you get in eight hours, you're going to be in good shape.

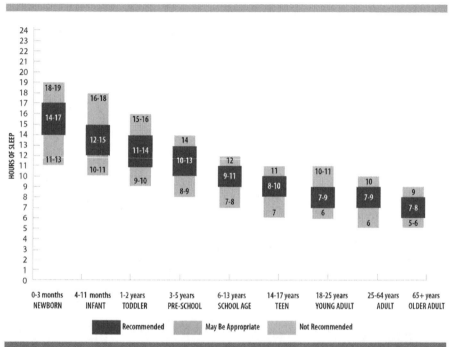

SLEEP DURATION RECOMMENDATIONS

Need Some Help Getting to Sleep?

1) GET UNPLUGGED

Turn off your electronics two hours before bedtime. Light can interfere with your sleep rhythms, but the blue light from electronics is especially distracting.

2) LIMIT CAFFEINE TO MORNING

Caffeine can affect you up to 12 hours after drinking it. Consider cutting back your daily intake.

3) AVOID LATE-NIGHT, HEAVY FOODS

It's okay to eat up until bedtime, but keep it light.

4) GET YOUR WATER IN EARLY

If you drink too much in the evening, you may end up making potty trips when you should be dreaming.

5) KEEP IT COOL

Most people sleep best in a cool room. Generally a temperature of about 65 degrees helps people sleep best.

6) SPLURGE FOR A GOOD BED

Make sure you have room to stretch and turn. If you wake up with a sore back, it's time to make a change.

W.A.I.T.*loss* Challenge:
Evaluate your sleep patterns, and make an individualized plan to get in eight hours of sleep each night.

Key #10: Preparation

What happens when you go to the grocery store without a list? If you're anything like me, you come home with a lot of TV dinners and mac-and-cheese. What happens if you get home late from work and haven't thought about dinner? If you're anything like me, you point your kids toward the TV dinners and mac-and-cheese. Although when I'm feeling I-suck-as-a-mom guilt, I stop and grab a pizza. (The tomato sauce counts as a vegetable . . . right?)

Preparation reduces willpower depletion. By being organized and prepared, we relieve the brain of having to keep track of everything. Lessening that load allows the PFC to have more strength to do other things, like resist the afternoon munchies. In other words, being organized preserves brain energy, which in turn relieves anxiety. (Less anxiety also means less cortisol, which means less stress weight gain.)

Does it seem like an impossible task to get prepared? It did to me, but you don't have to be perfect—any little effort will help. We are not born with an "organization" gene. It's something we need to cultivate and make into a habit. Here are some tips to help make it simple:

1) PUT THINGS DOWN ON PAPER

I have a notepad that I keep by my bed. Instead of staying up worrying about something I forgot to do, I write it down to remember the next day. This is immediate boss-brain relief and helps me get in my healthy sleep habit!

2) KEEP A CALENDAR

I used to write things down on little scrap papers all over the place. Needless to say, I missed a lot of appointments. Now my entire life is stored in the mysterious Internet cloud. I can access my schedule from multiple instruments at any time.

3) SHARE RESPONSIBILITIES

Isn't this why we have children? Delegating things like dinner and chores to them not only saves you time, it helps them learn and mature. Don't be afraid to let them help.

4) GET RID OF CLUTTER

I've been trying to teach this to my husband for almost 20 years. He likes to save everything. I try to sneak his cow-boyish things into the box on thrift store pick-up day, but he has a sixth sense and seems to find them every time. He has a deer-hoof gun rack that has been in and out of the giveaway box at least 100 times. Right now as I type, his piece of glossy shellacked wood with a rattlesnake skin is hanging in the garage waiting for me. In case saving your brain energy isn't enough reason to de-clutter, studies have found that when people eat in cluttered spaces, they end up eating more. In one study of 100 women, each was individually brought into one of two rooms: a messy kitchen or a tidy kitchen. The women were given a writing assignment and were told they could eat as many of the provided cookies as they wanted. Researchers found that the women in the cluttered kitchen ate twice as many cookies! **(2.25)** So if you haven't used it in a year, you probably don't need it. If you have used it, but it's worth less than a dollar, it's not worth the rent of the space it's taking up.

5) DON'T PUT THINGS OFF

If you're thinking that it needs to get done, go ahead and do it! If you do it while you're thinking about it, your PFC won't need to keep track.

6) MENTAL REHEARSAL

I first learned about mental rehearsal from Dave Blanchard, CEO of the Og Mandino Group. He is also my business coach and a good friend. Dave uses mental creation every day not only to plan but also to receive inspiration and vivid insight. Dave writes in his book, *Today I Begin a New Life*, "Success is created in two very different yet essential and complementary stages. The first stage is mental creation. The second is physical creation. Both are required. One does not occur without the other if we want our dreams to be realized in tangible reality." **(2.26)**

Mental creation also plays a big part in athletic training. Michael Jordan once remarked, "Basketball is more mental than physical." He said he would practice in his mind before the games to overcome his weaknesses. We can do this same thing in preparing for the day. The electrical activity produced in our minds is the same whether we are thinking about a task or actually performing it. For example, when Michael Jordan mentally rehearsed throwing a free throw, his brain reacted as if he had actually thrown it. **(2.27)**

If you take a few minutes to mentally rehearse your day, it can run a lot smoother. Mentally rehearse situations that might present themselves, such as a business lunch where you may have to decline dessert. If you can picture yourself performing the desired action in your mind before it happens, you are more likely to follow through when the situation arises.

7) HAVE ONE DAY A WEEK THAT YOU PREPARE THE WEEK'S MENU

You can write down recipes and make a shopping list from the week's menu you've made, or you can even prepare meals ahead of time and freeze them. I like to cut up vegetables and have them in a container, so they are easy to grab and munch on. Set them out after school, and I'll bet your kids will start to nibble as well.

8) CLEAR UNHEALTHY FOOD OUT OF YOUR HOUSE

I did my own study on visual food cues a while back. Soft caramel popcorn is my favorite food in the world. I could live off of it forever. I made some for my kids one night while they were watching a movie with friends (rookie mistake). I wrapped the leftover popcorn in plastic wrap and decided to leave it out in the open as a way to strengthen my willpower. I figured that if each resisted urge strengthened my boss-brain's willpower muscle, this caramel popcorn would surely give me lots of brain brawn quick! To make a long story short, it didn't work. It didn't even come close to working. I lasted 24 hours and then ate all of it in a one-night binge fest. So my recommendation to you is to not tempt fate. Get rid of the stuff that is going to make things more difficult for you. Acknowledging our urges and walking away *will* strengthen our self-control, but we don't all start off with biceps like Rosie the Riveter. Baby steps.

W.A.I.T. *loss* Challenge:
Wake up five minutes earlier
than you normally do. Use that
time to mentally rehearse your day
and what you want to accomplish.

Key #11: Support

I'm not listing support as a major Key to health because support what I do. I do it because *support* is a major Key to health! There are actually scientifically documented studies proving the importance of support in health and weight loss. **(2.28)**

One study followed 23 women 18 months after they had completed a weight-loss program. The women who maintained their weight indicated that the social support that they received was critical in their success. **(2.29, 2.30)**

Support can come from external sources as well as from internal sources. When I was married to my first husband, it was tough to be healthy. He wasn't unhealthy per se, but he did have a sweet tooth. He could eat whatever he wanted and stay thin. Unfortunately, I could not. It's pretty tough to not eat ice cream when your spouse is sitting next to you with a mouthful.

My current husband, on the other hand, is very careful about what he eats. He works out every day and is very health conscious. He would rather eat collard greens than a cookie, and chicken over pasta. I would rather eat dirt than collard greens, but it has been much easier for me to make good choices when I have a husband with the same goals.

My mom always told me that I needed to be careful about the friends I chose because I would more than likely end up just like them. Now that I'm a mom I see how true that is! My high school friends stayed away from drugs and alcohol. They went to college. They married and had kids. I did the exact same things. It's no different in respect to health. If you surround yourself with people who don't care about what they put in their mouths, you will more than likely be the same way. If you choose friends who choose health, you can pretty much bet that you will too.

If your friends and family seem to sabotage your good choices, there are other means of external support. Obviously I think the best is to have a wonderful health coach that can stand in your corner as well as help you with accountability. But other options include groups, such as Weight Watchers and Overeaters Anonymous. There are also a ton of social media and online groups that you can join. Many companies these days are also encouraging their employees to get healthy by offering weight-loss challenges and nutrition courses. If your work doesn't have a wellness program, maybe you can head one up!

Personally, I think having a higher-level "why" is more important than any external support. If you don't want to make a change in your life, it really doesn't matter how many other people want it for you. That's something that comes from within. Some people come by that naturally, and others obtain it the hard way—a diabetes diagnosis, a heart attack, an inability to get up from a chair. But however it happens, it's vital to any lasting changes.

Though I advocate personal responsibility for our choices and though I know from personal experience that I myself have control over my urges, I know for a fact that steps 2 and 3 of the Twelve-Step Program are for real. **(2.31)**

> *STEP 2.* Came to believe that a Power greater than our-
> selves could restore us to sanity.

STEP 3. Made a decision to turn our will and our lives
over to the care of God as we understood Him.

Generally speaking, addicts don't start out on their knees asking for help, but hitting rock bottom enough times will often put them there, even those who have never believed in a higher power. Eric Clapton was one of these. Unfortunately, his rock bottom didn't happen until after he had wrecked his marriage, hurt his career, and was contemplating suicide. He says of the experience:

> At that moment, almost of their own accord, my legs gave way and I fell to my knees. In the privacy of my room I begged for help. I had no notion who I thought I was talking to, I just knew that I had come to the end of my tether, I had nothing left to fight with. Then I remembered what I had heard about surrender, something I thought I could never do, my pride just wouldn't allow it, but I knew that on my own I wasn't going to make it, so I asked for help, and, getting down on my knees, I surrendered. **(2.32)**

He hasn't had a drink since then, not even when his baby boy fell 53 stories to his death.

How could turning yourself over to God have such dramatic results?

I've always been a religious person. I'm the first to admit that I'm worthless on my own. Fortunately, it's easy for me to get on my knees and ask for help. I couldn't have written this book without it. I have my own thoughts as to why believing in a higher power gives us more self-control.

Though faith is a hard thing for the scientific community to quantify, even agnostic scientists have to admit that it works. In Baumeister and

Tierney's book, *Willpower: Rediscovering the Greatest Human Strength,* they state that they are both agnostic but can't deny the data:

> We have no trouble believing there's some kind of power working at 12-Step meetings and religious services. Although many scientists are skeptical of institutions that promote spirituality—and psychologists, for some reason, have been particularly skeptical of religion—self-control researchers have developed a grudging respect for the practical results. **(2.33)**

In a series of experiments, researchers found that absolute religious concepts not only help people gain greater self-control, they also refuel people's ability to practice restraint. **(2.34)**

Finally, I think the best support you can receive comes through the support that you give others. In the program that I coach, we encourage people to "pay it forward" and teach others the things that they have learned. Not only does being an example help with personal accountability, by reaching outward, we can create our own circle of health. **(2.35)**

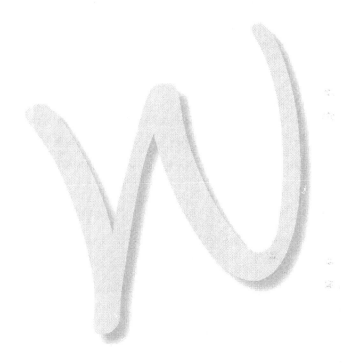

Section 3: W.A.I.T.
Putting It All Together

$Applying$ all of $these$ physical and mindful Keys had a huge impact on my health. I felt so much better than I ever had, but I still had times when The Brat's urges were too much to ignore. I knew my willpower was getting stronger as the binges, and even the urges to binge, were more spread out, but sometimes when I did fall back into bingeing, it was hard to crawl back out. I could go weeks without a binge, but then when I did succumb, it would be days before I could rein it in again. I felt at times like a drunk who couldn't stay on the wagon. As a matter of fact, I was *exactly* like a drunk. Only my addiction started with the conscious choice to eat a bag of candy. I wasn't sure when that choice to eat turned into an addiction, but an addiction it was. Understanding habit and addiction formation and the difference between the two was the final piece of the puzzle for me.

Actions to Habits, Habits to Addictions

All addictions start out as habits. All habits start out as actions. So in order to explain how one becomes addicted to food (or anything else), we must first explain how actions turn into habits.

Actions first happen in the adult part of the brain. When we start anything new, it requires thought (PFC duty). Think of the first time you had to tie your shoe. Whether you used the rabbit ears method or magic knot technique, it required deliberate effort and concentration. I'm guessing that by now, you can tie your shoes and think about what you're making for dinner at the same time, right? The reason you can tie your shoes with hardly any thought is because as you repeated the action over and over, there were neural pathways being created in the limbic region (The Brat) of your brain.

A neural pathway, or "Habit Loop," is like a scratch in a piece of wood. The more you "scratch" it, the deeper it gets. So once an action becomes a habit, it is no longer stored in the thinking part of your brain. It is stored in the limbic system. This is both good and not so good. Good because it frees up your PFC to learn new things. Not so good because it makes changing a bad habit difficult. Unless we make a deliberate and conscious effort, the bad habit will continue automatically, without much mental effort, especially if that habit has become an addiction.

A Habit Loop consists of three parts: 1) the cue (or trigger), 2) the routine, and 3) the reward. The trigger generally falls into one of the following categories: **(3.1)**

- Place
- Time
- Emotional state
- Person
- Preceding event

The routine is the action itself, and the reward is whatever makes the routine worth doing.

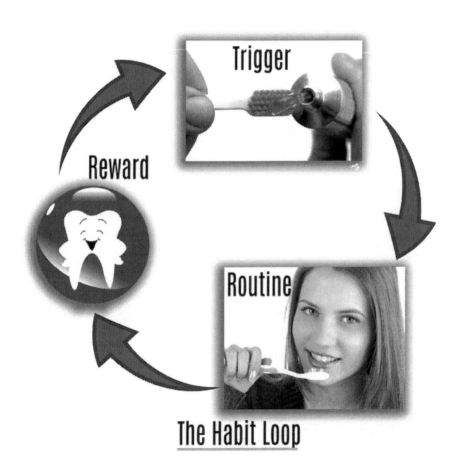

Starting a new habit is a lot easier than breaking an old one. Generally finding a good trigger can get a new Habit Loop up and running quickly. For example, if we need to get into the habit of brushing our teeth before bed, we can put a toothbrush on our pillow. Seeing the toothbrush will trigger the routine (brushing), and the reward will be less cavities and hopefully much better breath.

Breaking an old habit, on the other hand, is not so easy. You can't erase an existing Habit Loop anymore than you can rub out the scratch in the wood. The good news though is that a new "scratch" can be formed, and through neglect, the old "scratch" can be eventually forgotten. This type of behavioral treatment is called habit reversal training. The way that it works is to break down the Habit Loop and replace the unhealthy routine with a healthy one. The trigger and the reward stay the same.

Brad Dufrene, a psychologist who practices habit reversal training, calls the new routine a "competing response." One of Dufrene's patients was a girl who was a chronic nail-biter. She was not a typical case, however. She would bite until her nails were completely pulled from the skin. Her fingers were covered in scabs and showed signs of nerve damage.

Dufrene asked the patient to describe exactly what she was feeling before she put her hand to her mouth. She said it was anxiety, like a tension in her fingertips. Dufrene had her go home and carry around an index card. Each time she felt the cue (trigger)—the tension in her fingertips—he had her make a check mark on the index card. A week later she had 28 check marks on the card.

Dufrene then gave her the assignment to practice a competing response before putting her fingers in her mouth. She was to do something with her hands, such as grip a pencil or put her hands in her pockets. She was then to do anything that would produce a physical sensation, rub her arm or rap her knuckles on a desk, etc. In other words, the cues (tension) and the reward (physical stimulation) stayed the same. Only the routine was changed.

She was sent home with the assignment to continue with the index card but to make a check mark when she felt the tension and a hash mark when she circumvented the habit. The next week she had bitten her nails only three times. After a month, she was no longer biting her nails. She had replaced the bad routine with a competing one. **(3.2, 3.3)**

My Failed Attempt at Habit Reversal

Habit reversal training is typically used to treat people with tic disorders like nail-biting or skin-picking, but I hoped that I could also use it to overcome my bingeing. **(3.4)** I knew the first step was to identify my triggers, so I decided to apply Dufrene's technique and carry around an index card to track my urges. It was at this time that I came up with W.A.I.T. I was having a hard time slowing down enough to recognize my triggers, so I wanted a visual reminder. "What Am I Thinking" was a little long for my index card, so I just wrong down the first letters, W.A.I.T. Then every time I looked at it, I would try to stop and "hear" the thoughts in my mind. *Was I hungry? Was it a craving? If it was a craving, what was the trigger?* I started writing them down, and if I could tell the craving to go away, I gave myself a check mark. As far as self-awareness goes, the index card was working great. I was identifying my triggers and listening to my thoughts, but the competing response was still an issue.

Remember that in habit reversal training, the trigger and the reward stay the same. It's the routine that changes, and I couldn't seem to find a routine that worked for me. At first I decided to try some of the replacement routines that the "experts" recommended, taking a walk, listening to music, reading a book, knitting, etc. **(3.5, 3.6)** I realized fast that all of these things required too much effort. Bingeing was a lot easier and took less effort, or so it seemed.

I decided that I needed a simpler, effortless routine. I tried deep breathing, clenching my fists, push-ups on my kitchen counter. None of these things worked. None. By this time, I knew that I was getting closer to understanding the binge mystery, and I was a woman on a mission. I started reading whatever I could find on habits and addictions, and in my quest, I figured out where I had gone wrong. I didn't need *habit* reversal. I needed *addiction* reversal. I was trying to reconfigure a "Habit Loop," when I was dealing with an "Addiction Loop."

Habit Loop vs. Addiction (Broken) Loop

Addictions may start out as habits, but in the end, they are quite different. "Addiction Loops" are missing the best part of the Habit Loop—the reward. The reason drugs, alcohol, gambling, sex, food, etc., become addictions is because they cause dopamine to be released which, in turn, causes an intense reaction in a part of the brain called the pleasure center. The pleasure center is responsible for that euphoric feeling you get during pleasurable experiences, such as an orgasm.

Here's where the big problem lies. In the case of addictive substances, it's not actually the pleasure center that is activated. Addictions cause a reaction in another part of the brain that doesn't produce pleasure, but instead produces the *anticipation* of pleasure. In terms of the Habit Loop, it's not a reward. It's an *expectation* of a reward. That is the definition of a craving. It's the *desire* for something, *not* the something itself. To put it bluntly, addictions are like arousal with no climax. No matter how much an addict eats or drinks or gets high, there is no real satisfaction.

No wonder my competing responses weren't working! An "Addiction Loop" is a broken Habit Loop. Instead of being driven by a reward, it's driven by a craving. I realized that for "addiction reversal" I needed to replace not only the routine—I needed to find a reward.

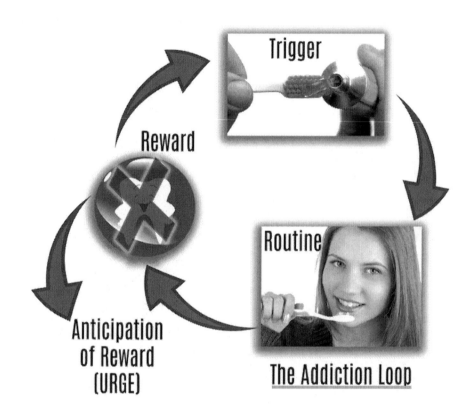

Trigger

Reward

Routine

Anticipation
of Reward
(URGE)

The Addiction Loop

The Reward (3.7, 3.8, 3.9)

Though they didn't work for me, the replacement routines could actually provide an appropriate reward. For example, if you binge because you are stressed, the reward should alleviate your stress. (Bingeing does the opposite!) Taking a walk, listening to music, yoga, etc., would probably be great stress relievers. The problem that I had with those was time. Most of my triggers were stress-related, and often I was stressed because I didn't have enough time to get things done. Routines like walking, yoga, etc., are too time-consuming to be realistic replacements for me.

I needed something quick and easy. I found a tally counter to help me keep track of how many cravings I ignored. Each time I resisted a craving, I gave myself a click on the counter. (I called it my Cravings Clicker.) My thought was to do something special for myself once I reached a certain number, but I never needed to do that. I'm not sure when or how it happened, but after a while, the click itself became the reward. Maybe it was because of the self-satisfaction that came with each individual click. Maybe it was some sensory thing. (I tried a counter that didn't *click*, and I didn't like it. I did need the *click* itself.) Or maybe a combination of both. But in any case, with W.A.I.T. serving as the routine and the click of the Cravings Clicker serving as the reward, I had started a new Habit Loop—one that directed me away from my food Addiction Loop.

The best part was I could almost feel my willpower strengthening each time I resisted an urge to binge. It was fun, too. It became a game of me against The Brat. I enjoyed keeping track of how many times I could ignore my urges, and it was really satisfying to look at the number on my Cravings Clicker and see how many "points" I had! Also, it took some time, but eventually the urges did begin to get quieter, and the space between them grew. Whereas I used to get ten clicks in a day, now I'm "lucky" to have ten in a month.

Keep in mind that even when a new Habit Loop is created, the old one is still lurking near, just waiting for the opportunity to take over again. So be patient with yourself, and understand that it's completely normal to fall back into old habits. Eventually, as long as you don't give up, your new Habit Loop will be your norm, and the Addiction Loop will be forgotten.

Another thing I noticed was that focusing on the urges I ignored, instead of those I didn't, meant no negativity sucking up my willpower reserves. I didn't have to beat myself up for bingeing anymore because I knew that eventually my willpower would be strong enough to resist. I just told myself that overeating was normal and gave myself a click for only having three bowls of ice cream instead of four.

To Restrict or Not to Restrict... That is the Question

I've read several opinions on whether people who binge should restrict themselves from eating trigger foods or not. Personally, I've found that if I tell myself I can't have something, it doesn't take long before I'm eating ten times the normal amount of that exact something. It's one of the great diet dilemmas. If we restrict, we binge. If we allow ourselves a taste, we still binge.

I've found it helpful to limit my trigger foods to earlier in the day when I know my willpower hasn't been depleted and my self-regulation is in full swing. If I know my willpower has been depleted, I try to stay away from temptation.

Another thing I have learned is that we can trick our brain into believing we are not restricting. A study done at the University of Chicago studied this phenomenon with three groups of basketball players. One group practiced foul shots for 30 days straight. The second group was told to "imagine" shooting foul shots for the same amount of time. Group three did nothing. They found that group three showed no improvement. Group one improved 24 percent, and group two improved 23 percent. **(3.10, 3.11)** The brain couldn't separate the real and the imagined.

The results of this study show just how greatly the brain can believe whatever we tell it. And I opt for using our brain's ability to believe to our own advantage. This is what I do: oftentimes when I want something that I know is a trigger for me, I'll tell myself that of course I can have it! But first I'm going to eat something healthy. Or first I'm going to go get the mail. Or first I'm going to put the laundry in the dryer— anything to get my mind in another direction for a minute. Before I know it, I've forgotten all about it. But the best part is that I don't feel deprived because I never told myself I couldn't.

When Leo Tolstoy was a boy he used to play a game where he had to stand in the corner until he could *not* think of a white bear. Leo always ended up staying in the corner for a long time because once told *not* to think of something, that's pretty much all anyone can think about. Kelly McGonigal explains the reasoning behind this in her book, *The Willpower Instinct: How Self-Control Works, Why It Matters, and What You Can Do to Get More of It*:

The problem with prohibition extends to any thought we try to ban. The latest research on anxiety, depression, dieting, and addiction all confirm: "I won't" power fails miserably when it's applied to the inner world of thoughts and feelings. **(3.12)**

It's for this reason that I don't say no to my urges. Instead I say to that part of my brain, "Sure. But in a moment—first I've got to take a nap (or eat something healthy, take a walk or you fill in the blank)."

All of this kind of reminds me of when my daughter asked me if she could have a monkey. Obviously, she wasn't going to be able to have a monkey, but I told her, "Sure. If you can find a monkey, you can have it." She was very happy and never asked me about it again. Had I told her no, I would have never heard the end of it. Treat the donuts like a monkey. Sure you can have it, just not this second. Then give yourself a click!

W.A.I.T.-and-Click Approach

It took a little time, but eventually my W.A.I.T.-card routine and click reward became habitual. I still wear my Cravings Clicker around my neck and often use it to help me stop at just a bite or two of something. The other day my daughter brought home a giant chocolate chip cookie. She left it in the kitchen, and I mindlessly took a bite. I started to go in for a second bite (which would inevitably lead to a third, fourth, and seventh), and then I remembered that if I resisted, I would get a click. I decided I would rather have a click than the cookie, so I walked away.

I make that choice 85 to 90 percent of the time. Sometimes I do choose to have a cookie (or two or three or five). But that's okay because it's normal to overeat every once in a while. The point is my willpower is much stronger than it used to be. Maybe eventually I'll decide to be a bodybuilder. If so, I'll have to be much stricter than I am now. But for the present, I'm at peace knowing that I have the power within myself to make that choice.

W.A.I.T.-and-Click at a Glance

I decided to put W.A.I.T.-and-Click into a simple step-by-step process so that it's easy to follow and apply. This technique was created to help me overcome my bingeing, but it can apply anytime you feel the need to ignore The Brat voice in your head.

Here are the things you will need:

- Index card
- Cravings Clicker (Anything that will keep track of your cravings will work. The one I like is available on my website.)
- Motivation to conquer The Brat

W.A.I.T. (Routine)

Step 1: On the front of an index card, write W.A.I.T.

Step 2: Below that write your higher level "why" (the driving force behind your motivation). Below is your Awareness Card, what you will use as a reminder to stop and "hear" the thoughts coming from The Brat.

W.A.I.T.

What am I thinking?

Why do I want to get healthy?

Higher Level "Why"

Step 3: On the back of the card, write *Time & Trigger, Acknowledge,* and *Ignore.*

Step 4: Keep the card in a place where you can see it often. When you do, stop and ask yourself, *"What Am I Thinking?"* If you are headed into the kitchen to binge, ask yourself if you are feeling hunger or a craving. If it's a craving, try to identify the trigger. Write it in the "Trigger" column.

Time & Trigger	Acknowledge	Ignore

Step 5: Take a second to acknowledge the craving. "Yes, urge, I hear you." Mark the "Acknowledge" column with a check mark.

Step 6: If you ignore the craving, mark it with a check mark.

Time & Trigger		Acknowledge	Ignore
3 pm	Fatigue	✓	✓
5 pm	Argue with kids		
10 am	Passed donut shop	✓	✓
9 pm	Watching movie	✓	✓

Cravings Clicker (Reward)*

Step 7: If you ignored the urge, give yourself a click on your Cravings
Clicker!

The Clicker Club

Before this book went to print, I decided that I needed to try the W.A.I.T.-and-Click Approach with others, as previously I had been the sole subject. I started a "Clicker Club" on Facebook for anyone who wanted to give it a try. The results were amazing! People started using their Cravings Clicker for bingeing as well as other times they resisted The Brat. One person even used it to help her clean her house. When she ignored The Brat's plea to procrastinate the chore, she gave herself a click. Another participant gave herself a click when she resisted spending money needlessly. My friend Brittany called me and said her son has been using it to not wash his hands (he has OCD, and it's working for him!). I know another person who is using it to resist the urge to smoke. My husband works from home where it's tough to avoid distractions. He decided to give himself a click for every day he stays on task. If he sticks to his schedule for ten days, he gives himself a day off. If you are interested in joining the Clicker Club, just go to my website (www. wendryhendry.com). I would *love* to hear how *you* are using your clicker.

Last Minute Reflections

My daughter, Hope, is an amazing competitive rock climber. Watching her pull herself up a rock with just her fingertips blows my mind. She has incredible strength. But she didn't start off climbing Everest. Should she beat herself up for that? Of course not! She celebrates each little advance. The self-evaluation at the beginning of the book can help you with that. Take it again in a year from now and monitor how far you've come.

If you only get one thing out of this book, I hope it's that same mindset. It is NOT all-or-nothing! You can and should celebrate the two steps forward. Don't worry about the one step back! That just means you're working toward Everest! The progress happens when you don't give up. The magic happens when you learn that the "one step back" is merely training grounds for growth. The more weaknesses, the more trials. The more trials, the more empathy. The more empathy, the better we can reach out and serve others.

It sure hasn't been an easy road, but I'm grateful for my persistent struggles with food. Had I been able to stop bingeing right after reading *Brain over Binge*, I would have missed out on learning so much more about mindfulness and habits and willpower. I would have missed helping those who needed a little more like I did!

> ## W.A.I.T. *loss* Challenge:
> My last challenge for you is to track your progress in a journal. Write down the things you have learned as well as the things you are still learning on your road to recovery. Then find others who are struggling and help them along the path. Here's one of my husband's favorite poems to inspire you along the way:

The Bridge Builder
By Will Allen Dromgoole

An old man going a lone highway,
Came, at the evening cold and gray,
To a chasm vast and deep and wide.
Through which was flowing a sullen tide
The old man crossed in the twilight dim,
The sullen stream had no fear for him;
But he turned when safe on the other side
And built a bridge to span the tide.

"Old man," said a fellow pilgrim near,
"You are wasting your strength with building here;
Your journey will end with the ending day,
You never again will pass this way;
You've crossed the chasm, deep and wide,
Why build this bridge at evening tide?"

The builder lifted his old gray head;
"Good friend, in the path I have come," he said,
"There followed after me to-day
A youth whose feet must pass this way.
This chasm that has been as naught to me
To that fair-haired youth may a pitfall be;
He, too, must cross in the twilight dim;
Good friend, I am building this bridge for him!" **(3.13)**

I hope this book will serve as a sturdy bridge to help you and other pilgrims cross the chasm to living the healthiest and most rewarding life possible. Keep in touch and don't forget to click!

Quotes from the Clicker Club

Today I gave myself a click just for choosing to USE my clicker today! Ha-ha. Today I'm clickin' away! Got through the grocery store successfully without anything "extra," so that was worth a few extra clicks for me!   —**Adrienne N.**

Sixteen clicks and feeling proud!   —**Larry C.**

Four today. Feeling so much more in control. Currently food doesn't own me. I make my choices and feel so incredible when I choose health.   —**Heidi R.**

I pretty much clicked all day long today. But I never caved—not once. Success!   —**Becky B.**

Three clicks. Caved once.   —**Jackie S.**

I forgot to prep my food last night, and this morning I was running late . . . and thought to myself, "I'll just get something from the vending machine." But then I WAIT-ed and prepped some carrots! I was late but totally worth it!   —**Claire P.**

I can feel that this approach is really helping me be mindful about my triggers. Each time I click, a little ounce of self-confidence trickles back into my being, helping me get it right more and more often.—**Jazlyn U.**

I am so grateful for the W.A.I.T. technique. Knowing my clicker was around my neck helped me get through an extremely emotional day.

—**Laura A.**

I made homemade mac-n-cheese for the family tonight. I made myself homemade cauliflower and cheese! Low-fat cheese and all! It was the BOMB! Three clicks today.

—**Shauna K.**

Ten times today!! I am also having less urges and made great choices with my food. I am definitely being more mindful with my eating since I started this!

—**Trish J.**

Today I used my clicker 14 times—it was a rough day, but I made it. There were times I didn't have my clicker with me, but I would just W.A.I.T. and then say "click."

—**Teralyn S.**

Acknowledgments

I used to think acknowledgments at the end of books were just for sycophants. But after writing this book, I realize the error of my ways. The material has come as much or more from others as it has from my own experience, and I feel rather guilty that their names are not listed with mine on the cover. This book would have never happened without my team of health coaches who have become my family. I would rather walk this path with them than any others in the whole world. Also, I have coached the most amazing people who have taught me much more than I could have ever taught them. This book was written for my favorite clients . . . all 1,061 of them.

Thank you to my special pre-editors: Rillene Nielson, Bobbi Frampton, Shalisa Goates, and Renee Slater (thanks for the "lube" analogy!). Thanks to my friend Victoria Vigil who talked me into writing in the first place and my accountibilibuddy, Davina Chessid. Thank you to all of my mentors Dr. Wayne Anderson, Dan Bell, Kim Fiske, Jared and Amber Smithson, especially Shantelle Flake who gave me the confidence that my ramblings may actually help someone. Thanks to my beautiful Fempresses for their help and encouragement, and all of my wonderful Facebook friends whose opinions I value so much.

I want to thank those who worked as hard as I did to get this book launched. Thanks to Nancy Pile, my editor, Ida Sveningsson, who designed the awesome cover, Karen Christoffersen and Dayna Linton my cool producers at Bookwise Publishing and the most patient women in the world. Also to Aron Benon, the guys at meltdownchallenge.com and Emily Peterson at the Magnolia Agency for my fabulous website. I'm grateful to my SPS group and especially my coach Ramy Vance who wouldn't let me rest until I finished. To Alex Valente with alexvalente-photography.com for all his wonderful photographs.

I want to thank my parents . . . all five of them, for not only giving me life but for loving me and for making me believe that I can do anything. Eddy, for giving me Jewish genes that I'm proud to carry. Jan, for giving me good hair and strong legs and for being a hot grandma. John, for putting up with me (and my crazy family) and providing me the "cool factor" of saying my dad makes guns for the military. And especially to Janeen and Wendell for lying to me and telling me that I had a genius IQ. I know now that I don't but believing that I did carried me far. You were the best mom and dad in the world, and I miss you every single day.

Lastly, a very special thanks to my husband and kids who had to fend for themselves for four months while I stayed in my cave to write. I love you, Ron, Chris, Sarah, Trey, Chase, Declan, Rob, Cerani, Kale, Julianna, Xander, Kaity, Mateo, Claudia, Ryan, Tyler, Hope, and Chloe. I wouldn't change one thing about us.

Let me conclude by saying, I know it's not politically correct to talk about God and Jesus and faith, but I would be lying to you if I said I did this on my own. The Lord played the biggest part of all in my journey and He continues to. The best advice I could give you as you struggle through this or any trial is to get on your knees, picture a loving Father in your mind, and start asking for His help. He wants you to be happy even more than you want you to be happy.

Recommended Reading

Also, I have learned much of what I know from reading books written by people much smarter than me, and I want to make sure they are given credit here as well as in the citations. I wrote this list not only as a thank you to them, but also as a reference of books that I highly recommend.

- **Kathryn Hansen's** *Brain over Binge: Why I Was Bulimic, Why Conventional Therapy Didn't Work, and How I Recovered for Good*
- **Kathryn Hansen's** *The Brain over Binge Recovery Guide*
- **Wayne Scott Anderson's** *Habits of Health*
- **Wayne Scott Anderson's** *Discover Your Optimal Health*
- **Dave Blanchard's** *Today I Begin a New Life: Og Mandino for the 21st Century*
- **Dave Blanchard's** *The Observer's Chair: The Miracle of Healing Self Esteem*
- **Gordon S. Bruin's** *Language of Recovery: Understanding and Treating Addiction*
- **Jack Trimpey's** *Rational Recovery: The New Cure for Substance Addiction*
- **Kelly McGonigal's** *The Willpower Instinct*
- **Roy F. Baumeister's** and **John Tierney's** *Willpower: Rediscovering the Greatest Human Strength*
- **Charles Duhig's** *The Power of Habit*
- **Roy F. Baumeister's** and **John Tierney's** *Willpower: Rediscovering the Greatest Human Strength*

Reference Notes

0.1 "Institute for Health Metrics and Evaluation." Institute for Health Metrics and Evaluation. http://www.healthdata.org/.

0.2 "Obesity and Overweight." World Health Organization. http://www.who.int/mediacentre/factsheets/fs311/en/.

0.3 *National Health and Nutrition Examination Survey, Which Is Conducted by the Centers for Disease Control and Prevention.*

0.4 "Press Briefing Transcript." Centers for Disease Control and Prevention. May 7, 2012. http://www.cdc.gov/media/releases/2012/t0507_weight_nation.html.

0.5 "Navy SEALs: The Past, Present and Future of Unconventional Warfare." Navy SEALs. http://www.navyseals.com/.

0.6 Baumeister, Roy F., and John Tierney. *Willpower: Rediscovering the Greatest Human Strength.* New York: Penguin Press, 2011.

1.1 "Why I Suck at Intuitive Eating." ED Bites. July 12, 2013. http://edbites.com/2013/07/why-i-suck-at-intuitive-eating/.

1.2 Koch, Anne, and Olga Pollatos. "Interoceptive Sensitivity, Body Weight and Eating Behavior in Children: A Prospective Study." *Frontiers in Psychology Front. Psychol.* 5 (September 9, 2014).

1.3 "Meal Frequency & Weight Loss." Www.ideafit.com. July 28, 2008. http://www.ideafit.com/fitness-library/meal-frequency-weight-loss.

1.4 Benardot, Dan. *Nutrition for Serious Athletes.* Champaign, IL: Human Kinetics, 2000.

1.5 Fábry, P., Z. Hejl, J. Fodor, T. Braun, and Kamila Zvolánková. "The Frequency of Meals Its Relation To Overweight, Hypercholesterolæmia, And Decreased Glucose-Tolerance." *The Lancet* 284, no. 7360 (September 18, 1964): 614–15.

1.6 Thank you, Facebook and Fempresses!

1.7 Fábry, P., J. Fodor, Z. Hejl, Helena Geizerová, and Olga Balcarová. "Meal Frequency and Ischæmic Heart-Disease." *The Lancet* 292, no. 7561 (July 1968): 190–91.

1.8 Levitsky, David A., and Carly Pacanowski. "Losing Weight without Dieting. Use of Commercial Foods as Meal Replacements for Lunch Produces an Extended Energy Deficit." *Appetite* 57, no. 2 (October 2011): 311.

1.9 Schlundt D.G., J.O. Hill, T. Sbrocco, J. Pope-Cordle, and T. Sharp. "The role of breakfast in the treatment of obesity: a randomized clinical trial." *American Journal of Clinical Nutrition* 55, no. 3 (March 1992): 645–51.

1.10 Cahill, L.E., S.E. Chiuve, and R.A. Mekary. "Prospective Study of Breakfast Eating and Incident Coronary Heart Disease in a Cohort of Male US Health Professionals." *Journal of Vascular Surgery* 59, no. 2 (September 2012): 555.

1.11 "The Science Behind Breakfast." Rush University Medical Center. https://www.rush.edu/health-wellness/discover-health/why-you-should-eat-breakfast.

1.12 Enos, Deborah. "Four Reasons Why You Should Never Skip Breakfast" *Live Science*, September 12, 2013.

1.13 Daly, Annie. "Seven Reasons You NEED to Eat Carbs." *Women's Health*, August 21, 2014.

1.14 Benardot, Dan. *Nutrition for Serious Athletes.* Champaign, IL: Human Kinetics, 2000.

1.15 Arentson-Lantz, Emily, Stephanie Clairmont, Douglas Paddon-Jones, Angelo Tremblay, and Rajavel Elango. "Protein: A Nutrient in Focus 1." *Applied Physiology, Nutrition, and Metabolism* 40, no. 8 (2015): 755–61.

1.16 Bailey, Lydia. "Study: How Much Protein Do You Need?" *Men's Health*, July 23, 2015

1.17 Leech, Joe. "Why Are Trans Fats Bad For You? The Disturbing Truth", *Authority Nutrition*, July, 2015

1.18 Siri-Tarino, P. W., Q. Sun, F. B. Hu, and R. M. Krauss. "Meta-analysis of Prospective Cohort Studies Evaluating the Association of Saturated Fat with Cardiovascular Disease." *American Journal of Clinical Nutrition* 91, no. 3 (2010): 535–46.

1.19 "Heartorg Home Page." American Heart Association. Accessed March 25, 2016. http://www.heart.org/.

1.20 "About the Seven Countries Study." Seven Countries Study: The First Study to Relate Diet with Cardiovascular Disease. 1952. http://www.sevencountriesstudy.com/about-the-study/.

1.21 "Dodd-Frank Wall Street Reform 275 in the Last Year." *Federal Register.* June 17, 2015. https://www.federalregister.gov/articles/2015/06/17/2015-14883/final-determination-regarding-partially-hydrogenated-oils.

1.22 *Dietary Guidelines for Americans 2010.* Report.

1.23 Wansink, Brian, James E. Painter, and Jill North. "Bottomless Bowls: Why Visual Cues of Portion Size May Influence Intake." *Obesity Research* 13, no. 1 (January 2005): 93–100.

1.24 Rolls, Barbara J., Liane S. Roe, Tanja V.E. Kral, Jennifer S. Meengs, and Denise E. Wall. "Increasing the Portion Size of a Packaged Snack Increases Energy Intake in Men and Women." *Appetite* 42, no. 1 (December 2004): 63–69.

1.25 *Dietary Guidelines for Americans 2010.* Report.

1.26 "Ask the Dietitian® Home." Ask the Dietitian® Home. http://www.dietitian.com/.

1.27 "Holiday Strategies for Weight Loss—Dr. Wayne Andersen." Dr Wayne Andersen. December 22, 2013. http://www.drwayneandersen.com/2013/11/22/holiday-strategies-for-weight-loss-2/.

1.28 Pontzer, Herman, Ramon Durazo-Arvizu, Lara R. Dugas, Jacob Plange-Rhule, Pascal Bovet, Terrence E. Forrester, Estelle V. Lambert, Richard S. Cooper, Dale A. Schoeller, and Amy Luke. "Constrained Total Energy Expenditure and Metabolic Adaptation to Physical Activity in Adult Humans." *Current Biology* 26, no. 3 (2016): 410–17.

1.29 "Too Much Exercise Surprisingly Won't Result in Weight Loss—Study." RT International. https://www.rt.com/news/330622-exercise-weight-loss-obesity/.

1.30 Rosenbaum, M., and R. L. Leibel. "Adaptive Thermogenesis in Humans." *International Journal of Obesity* 34 (October 2010): 759–64.

1.31 "Does Cardio Make You Fat?" Poliquin—Healthy. Lean. Strong. March 3, 2014. http://main.poliquingroup.com/ArticlesMultimedia/Articles/Article/1138/Does_Cardio_Make_You_Fat.aspx.

1.32 http://www.medscape.com/viewarticle/567126_2

1.33 Brynjar Foss, Lars Rune Sæterdal, and Sindre M. Dyrstad. "Weight Reduction in Obese Correlates with Low Morning Cortisol Increase." *Journal of Exercise Physiology* 17, no. 3 (June 2014).

1.34 Mitch D. VanBruggen, Anthony C. Hackney, Robert G. McMurray, and Kristin S. Ondrak. "The Relationship between Serum and Salivary Cortisol Levels in Response to Different Intensities of Exercise." *International Journal of Sports Physiology and Performance*, no. 3 (September 6, 2011): 396–407.

1.35 "The Relationship Between Serum and Salivary Cortisol Levels in Response to Different Intensities of Exercise." Research Gate. July 13, 2014. https://www.researchgate.net/publication/51632095_The_Relationship_Between_Serum_and_Salivary_Cortisol_Levels_in_Response_to_Different_Intensities_of_Exercise.

1.36 "Is 'Starvation Mode' Real or Imaginary? A Critical Look." RSS 20. July 2015. http://authoritynutrition.com/starvation-mode/.

1.37 Marks, Bonita L., Ann Ward, Diane H. Morris, John Castellani, and James M. Rippe. "Fat-free Mass Is Maintained in Women following a Moderate Diet and Exercise Program.'" *Medicine and Science in Sports and Exercise* 27, no. 9 (September 1995).

1.38 "Lift to Lose Weight." Experience Life. September 01, 2012. https://experiencelife.com/article/lift-to-lose-weight/.

1.39 Manninen, Anssi H. "Very-low-carbohydrate Diets and Lean Body Mass." *Obesity Reviews* 7, no. 3 (2006): 297.

1.40 "Science Says Cheat Meals Actually Help You Lose Weight." Medical Daily. 2015 http://www.medicaldaily.com/9010-rule-cheat-meals-actually-boost-your-metabolism-and-help-you-lose-weight-327212.

1.41 "Exercise and Depression." Harvard Health. June 9, 2009. Accessed March 25, 2016. http://www.health.harvard.edu/mind-and-mood/exercise-and-depression-report-excerpt.

1.42 Chaddock-Heyman, Laura, Kirk I. Erickson, Joseph L. Holtrop, Michelle W. Voss, Matthew B. Pontifex, Lauren B. Raine, Charles H. Hillman, and Arthur F. Kramer. "Aerobic Fitness Is Associated with Greater White Matter Integrity in Children." *Frontiers in Human Neuroscience.* 8 (2014).

1.43 "Does Exercise Grow New Brain Cells?" *ACE Fitness*. November 4, 2011. https://www. acefitness.org/blog/2055/does-exercise-grow-new-brain-cells.

1.44 "Study: Exercise Can Boost Low Sex Drive Linked to Antidepressants." *UNews*. February 14, 2014. Accessed March 25, 2016. http://unews.ca/exercise_boost_sex_drive/.

1.45 White, James R., David A. Case, D. Mcwhirter, and A. M. Mattison. "Enhanced Sexual Behavior in Exercising Men." *Archives of Sexual Behavior* 19, no. 3 (1990): 193–209.

1.46 Ho, Suleen S., Satvinder S. Dhaliwal, Andrew P. Hills, and Sebely Pal. "The Effect of 12 Weeks of Aerobic, Resistance or Combination Exercise Training on Cardiovascular Risk Factors in the Overweight and Obese in a Randomized Trial." *BMC Public Health* 12, no. 1 (March 25, 2012): 704.

1.47 "Cortisol in Concurrent Training." Cortisol in Concurrent Training. https://www.unm. edu/~lkravitz/Article folder/cortisol.html.

1.48 Tyagi, Anupama, Marc Cohen, John Reece, and Shirley Telles. "An Explorative Study of Metabolic Responses to Mental Stress and Yoga Practices in Yoga Practitioners, Non-yoga Practitioners and Individuals with Metabolic Syndrome." *BMC Complementary and Alternative Medicine* 14, no. 1 (November 15, 2014): 445.

1.49 Okonta, Nkechi Rose. "Does Yoga Therapy Reduce Blood Pressure in Patients With Hypertension?" *Holistic Nursing Practice* 26, no. 3 (May/June 2012): 137–41.

1.50 Ross, Alyson, and Sue Thomas. "The Health Benefits of Yoga and Exercise: A Review of Comparison Studies." *The Journal of Alternative and Complementary Medicine* 16, no. 1 (2010): 3–12.

1.51 Cheung, Corjena, Juyoung Park, and Jean F. Wyman. "Effects of Yoga on Symptoms, Physical Function, and Psychosocial Outcomes in Adults with Osteoarthritis." *American Journal of Physical Medicine and Rehabilitation* 95, no. 2 (February 2016): 139–51.

1.52 Palmer, S. C., G. Wong, S. Iff, J. Yang, V. Jayaswal, J. C. Craig, E. Rochtchina, P. Mitchell, J. J. Wang, and G. F. M. Strippoli. "Fluid Intake and All-cause Mortality, Cardiovascular Mortality and Kidney Function: A Population-based Longitudinal Cohort Study." *Nephrology Dialysis Transplantation* 29, no. 7 (August 07, 2013): 1377–384.

1.53 ScienceDaily. February 4, 2004. https://www.sciencedaily.com/releases/2004/02/040212092439.htm.

1.54 "Clinical Trial Confirms Effectiveness of Simple Appetite Control Method." American Chemical Society. August 23, 2010. http://www.acs.org/content/acs/en/pressroom/newsreleases/2010/august/clinical-trial-confirms-effectiveness-of-simple-appetite-control-method.html.

1.55 Boschmann, Michael, Jochen Steiniger, Uta Hille, Jens Tank, Frauke Adams, Arya M. Sharma, Susanne Klaus, Friedrich C. Luft, and Jens Jordan. "Water-Induced Thermogenesis." *The Journal of Clinical Endocrinology and Metabolism* 88, no. 12 (2003): 6015–019.

1.56 Adan, Ana. "Cognitive Performance and Dehydration." *Journal of the American College of Nutrition* 31, no. 2 (April 12, 2012): 71–78.

1.57 "Drinking Water Improves Exam Grades, Research Suggests." BBC News. April 18, 2012. http://www.bbc.com/news/education-17741653.

1.58 Chan, J. "Water, Other Fluids, and Fatal Coronary Heart Disease: The Adventist Health Study." *American Journal of Epidemiology* 155, no. 9 (January 11, 2002): 827–33.

1.59 Pross, Nathalie, Agnès Demazières, Nicolas Girard, Romain Barnouin, Déborah Metzger, Alexis Klein, Erica Perrier, and Isabelle Guelinckx. "Effects of Changes in Water Intake on Mood of High and Low Drinkers." *PLoS ONE* 9, no. 4 (2014).

1.60 Blau, Joseph N., Christian A. Kell, and Julia M. Sperling. "Water-Deprivation Headache: A New Headache with Two Variants-A Response." *Headache: The Journal of Head and Face Pain* 44, no. 10 (January 2004): 1056–057.

1.61 Blau, Joseph N. "Water Deprivation: A New Migraine Precipitant." *Headache: The Journal of Head and Face Pain* 45, no. 6 (June 2005): 757–59.

1.62 "Thirty-four Proven Ways Water Makes You Better in Every Way." *Greatist.* January 6, 2015. http://greatist.com/health/health-benefits-water.

1.63 "Clinical Trial Confirms Effectiveness of Simple Appetite Control Method." American Chemical Society. August 23, 2010. Accessed March 26, 2016. http://www.acs.org/content/acs/en/pressroom/newsreleases/2010/august/clinical-trial-confirms-effectiveness-of-simple-appetite-control-method.html.

2.1 "An Irishman's Diary." *The Irish Times.* February 9, 2012. http://www.irishtimes.com/opinion/an-irishman-s-diary-1.460146.

2.2 Hansen, Kathryn. *Brain over Binge: Why I Was Bulimic, Why Conventional Therapy Didn't Work, and How I Recovered for Good.* (pp. 82–83) Phoenix, AZ: Camellia Publishing, 2011.

2.3 "Chapter 9—Limbic System." Chapter 9: Limbic System. https://www.dartmouth.edu/~rswenson/NeuroSci/chapter_9.html.

2.4 HowStuffWorks. http://science.howstuffworks.com/life/inside-the-mind/emotions/laughter4.htm.

2.5 Trimpey, Jack. *Rational Recovery: The New Cure for Substance Addiction.* New York: Pocket Books, 1996.

2.6 Trimpey, Jack. *Rational Recovery: The New Cure for Substance Addiction.* (ch. 12) New York: Pocket Books, 1996.

2.7 Hansen, Kathryn. *Brain over Binge: Why I Was Bulimic, Why Conventional Therapy Didn't Work, and How I Recovered for Good.* (p. 86) Phoenix, AZ: Camellia Publishing, 2011.

2.8 Baumeister, Roy F., and John Tierney. *Willpower: Rediscovering the Greatest Human Strength.* New York: Penguin Press, 2011.

2.9 "How Willpower Works." *Boston Globe.* November 7, 2011. https://www.bostonglobe.com/lifestyle/health-wellness/2011/11/07/how-willpower-works/XlOvEG4FipvZ8vM-8VUNBpK/story.html.

2.10 Danziger, S., J. Levav, and L. Avnaim-Pesso. "Extraneous Factors in Judicial Decisions." *Proceedings of the National Academy of Sciences* 108, no. 17 (February 11, 2011): 6889–892.

2.11 Cynkar, A. "Low Glucose Levels Compromise Self-control." *PsycEXTRA Dataset*, April 07.

2.12 Gailliot, M. T., and R. F. Baumeister. "The Physiology of Willpower: Linking Blood Glucose to Self-Control." *Personality and Social Psychology Review* 11, no. 4 (November 0 2007): 303-27.

2.13 Mergenthaler, Philipp, Ute Lindauer, Gerald A. Dienel, and Andreas Meisel. "Sugar for the Brain: The Role of Glucose in Physiological and Pathological Brain Function." *Trends in Neurosciences* 36, no. 10 (October 2013): 587-97.

2.14 Nixon, By Robin. "Brain Food: How to Eat Smart." LiveScience. January 07, 2009. http://www.livescience.com/3186-brain-food-eat-smart.html.

2.15 "Bad News: The Sugar Cravings Around Your Period Are Actually Ageing You." The Huffington Post UK. October 9, 14. http://www.huffingtonpost.co.uk/antonia-mariconda/sugar-cravings-period_b_5577578.html.

2.16 Tierney, John. "Do You Suffer From Decision Fatigue?" *The New York Times.* August 17, 2011. http://www.nytimes.com/2011/08/21/magazine/do-you-suffer-from-decision-fatigue.html?pagewanted=print.

2.17 "Meditation 101: Techniques, Benefits & Beginner's How-to." How to Meditate: Meditation Techniques, Benefits & Beginner's How-to. July 31, 31. http://life.gaiam.com/article/meditation-101-techniques-benefits-beginner-s-how.

2.18 Bruin, Gordon S. *The Language of Recovery: A Christian Perspective: Understanding & Treating Addiction.* S.I.: Gordon S. Bruin, 2010.

2.19 "Harvard Study Unveils What Meditation Literally Does To The Brain." Collective Evolution RSS. December 11, 2014. Accessed March 26, 2016. http://www.collective-evolution.com/2014/12/11/harvard-study-unveils-what-meditation-literally-does-to-the-brain/.

2.20 "Less Sleep Leads to More Eating and More Weight Gain, According to New CU-Boulder Study." News Center. March 11, 2013. http://www.colorado.edu/news/releases/2013/03/11/less-sleep-leads-more-eating-and-more-weight-gain-according-new-cu-boulder#sthash.CGKUzui0.dpuf.

2.21 Spiegel, Karine. "Brief Communication: Sleep Curtailment in Healthy Young Men Is Associated with Decreased Leptin Levels, Elevated Ghrelin Levels, and Increased Hunger and Appetite." *Annals of Internal Medicine* 141, no. 11 (December 07, 2004): 846.

2.22 Wikipedia contributors, "Leptin," *Wikipedia, The Free Encyclopedia*, https://en.wikipedia.org/w/index.php?title=Leptin&oldid=705426727.

2.23 Bailey, Bruce W., Matthew D. Allen, James D. Lecheminant, Larry A. Tucker, William K. Errico, William F. Christensen, and Marshall D. Hill. "Objectively Measured Sleep Patterns in Young Adult Women and the Relationship to Adiposity." *American Journal of Health Promotion* 29, no. 1 (September/October 2014): 46–54.

2.24 Digital image. https://sleepfoundation.org/sites/default/files/STREPchanges_1.png.

2.25 Vartanian, Lenny R., Kristen Kernan, and Brian Wansink. "Clutter, Chaos, and Over-consumption: The Role of Mind-Set in Stressful and Chaotic Food Environments." *SSRN Electronic Journal*, January 6, 2016.

2.26 Blanchard, Dave. *Today I Begin a New Life: Og Mandino for the 21st Century* (Kindle Location 314). Og Press. Kindle Edition. 2010.

2.27 "Mental Rehearsal." Mental Rehearsal. http://www.wright.edu/~scott.williams/Leader-Letter/rehearsal.htm.

2.28 "How Social Support Can Help You Lose Weight." APA org. http://www.apa.org/topics/obesity/support.aspx.

2.29 "News Bureau—ILLINOIS." News Bureau—ILLINOIS. https://news.illinois.edu/blog/view/6367/204477.

2.30 Metzgar, C. J., A. G. Preston, D. L. Miller, and S. M. Nickols-Richardson. "Facilitators and Barriers to Weight Loss and Weight Loss Maintenance: A Qualitative Exploration." *Journal of Human Nutrition and Dietetics* 28, no. 6 (September 18, 2014): 593–603.

2.31 *THE TWELVE STEPS OF ALCOHOLICS ANONYMOUS.*

2.32 Clapton, Eric. *Clapton: The Autobiography* (Kindle Locations 3502–3505). Crown/Archetype. Kindle Edition, 2007.

2.33 Baumeister, Roy F., and John Tierney. *Willpower: Rediscovering the Greatest Human Strength*. New York: Penguin Press, 2011.

2.34 "Rounding, K., A. Lee, J. A. Jacobson, and L.-J. Ji. "Religion Replenishes Self-Control." *Psychological Science* 23, no. 6 (June 11, 2012): 635–42.

2.35 Andersen, Wayne Scott. *Living a Longer Healthier Life: The Companion Guide to Dr. A's Habits of Health*. Annapolis, MD: Habits of Health Press, 2009.

3.1 Duhigg, Charles. *The Power of Habit: Why We Do What We Do in Life and Business*. New York: Random House, 2012.

3.2 Azrin, N. H., and R. G. Nunn, "Habit-Reversal: A Method of Eliminating Nervous Habits and Tics," Duhigg, Charles. *The Power of Habit: Why We Do What We Do in Life and Business* (Kindle Locations 4951–4952). Random House Publishing Group. Kindle Edition, 2012.

3.3 Dufrene, B. A., T. Steuart Watson, and J. S. Kazmerski. "Functional Analysis and Treatment of Nail Biting." *Behavior Modification* 32, no. 6 (November 09, 2008): 913–27.

3.4 Sayar, Gokben, and Gaye Kagan. "Habit Reversal Training in Trichotillomania: A Case Report." The Journal of Neurobehavioral Sciences 1, no. 1 (Winter 2012): 17.

3.5 "Ten Things To DO Instead of Binge Eating." HealthStatus. https://www.healthstatus.com/health_blog/health_tips/ten-things-to-do-instead-of-binge-eating/.

3.6 "Thin Intentions." Things to Do Instead of Eating. http://thinintentionsforever.blogspot.com/p/things-to-do-instead-of-eating_18.html.

3.7 Berridge, Kent C., and Morten L. Kringelbach. "Affective Neuroscience of Pleasure: Reward in Humans and Animals." *Psychopharmacology* 199, no. 3 (August 03, 2008): 457–80.

3.8 Schultz, Wolfram. "Behavioral Theories and the Neurophysiology of Reward." *Annual Review of Psychology* 57, no. 1 (September 16, 2005): 87–115.

3.9 McGonigal, Kelly. *The Willpower Instinct: How Self-Control Works, Why It Matters, and What You Can Do to Get More of It* (p. 210). Penguin Publishing Group. Kindle Edition, 2011.

3.10 "Mental Imagery in Sports Psychology." Sports Psychology for Peak Performance. http://www.sports-psychology.com/mental-imagery-in-sports-psychology/.

3.11 "Real or Imagined? The Brain Doesn't Know!" New Hope Outreach. 2008. https://newhopeoutreach.wordpress.com/related-articles/recovery-from-abuse/healing-emotional-memories/real-or-imagined-the-brain-doesnt-know/.

3.12 McGonigal, Kelly. *The Willpower Instinct: How Self-Control Works, Why It Matters, and What You Can Do to Get More of It* (p. 210). Penguin Publishing Group. Kindle Edition, 2011.

3.13 Greenberg, Arielle. "The Bridge Builder." Poetry Foundation. http://www.poetryfoundation.org/poem/237102.

About the Author

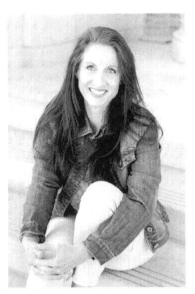

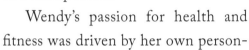 of the most inspiring women in the fitness industry. As well as being a fitness instructor and owner of Sweaty Chix Fitness™, she has motivated people in her role as a health and wellness coach and entrepreneur.

Wendy's passion for health and fitness was driven by her own personal struggle with food addiction and obesity. In her personal pursuit of health and healing, she began on a journey that would eventually strike a flame in thousands of women to get active. Ultimately becoming a certified Health Coach, she has been able to influence thousands more to overcome food addictions and unhealthy habits.

Wendy received her bachelor's degree in microbiology from Brigham Young University and is co-founder of Biolynk Corporation, an antibody recruitment company.

She currently lives with her family in the beautiful mountain community of Mapleton, Utah. When she's not helping clients or at the gym with her husband, she can be found reading Jane Austen, contemplating the amazing blessings that God has given her, and arguing politics with her children.

To purchase a Cravings Clicker and join the Clicker Club, or for more information on the nutrition program recommended by Wendy, visit her website at www.WendyHendry.com.

Look for more books from Wendy Hendry in the future.

Keep up to date with all the lastest information on Wendy's website:

www.WendyHendry.com.